CW00486756

Adele Glenn

INTERMITTENT FASTING
COOKBOOK:

Easy And Tasty Recipes For Your Healthy
Intermittent Fasting (Includes Keto Recipes)

© Copyright 2020 - All rights reserved.

The content contained within this book may not be reproduced, duplicated or transmitted without direct written permission from the author or the publisher.

Under no circumstances will any blame or legal responsibility be held against the publisher, or author, for any damages, reparation, or monetary loss due to the information contained within this book. Either directly or indirectly.

Legal Notice:

This book is copyright protected. This book is only for personal use. You cannot amend, distribute, sell, use, quote or paraphrase any part, or the content within this book, without the consent of the author or publisher.

Disclaimer Notice:

Please note the information contained within this document is for educational and entertainment purposes only. All effort has been executed to present accurate, up to date, and reliable, complete information. No warranties of any kind are declared or implied. Readers acknowledge that the author is not engaging in the rendering of legal, financial, medical or professional advice. The content within this book has been derived from various sources. Please consult a licensed professional before attempting any techniques outlined in this book.

By reading this document, the reader agrees that under no circumstances is the author responsible for any losses, direct or indirect, which are incurred as a result of the use of information contained within this document, including, but not limited to, errors, omissions, or inaccuracies.

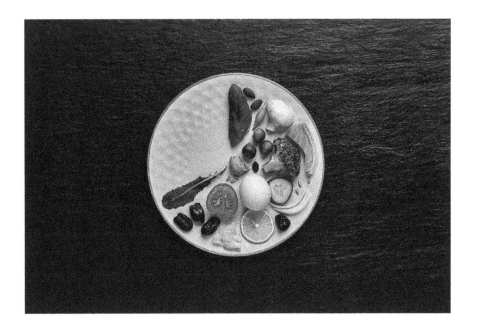

Table of Contents

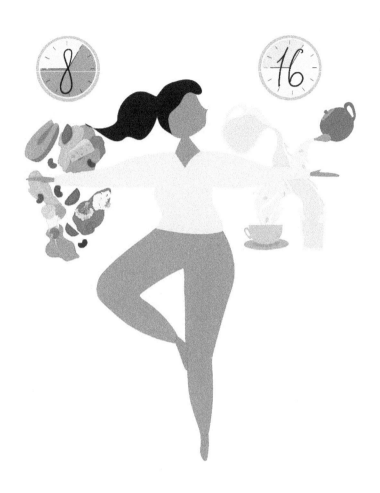

Introduction

Congratulations on purchasing your copy of *Intermittent Fasting*, and thank you for doing so. The following pages will provide you with the groundwork that will be essential for success using the ketogenic diet plan. Before you begin the journey to ketosis, here is a bit of insight on how the diet plan was discovered.

During the era of the 1920s and 1930s, the ketogenic diet was prevalent for its role in epilepsy therapy treatments. The diet plan provided a method other than the uncharacteristic techniques of fasting, which were popular in the treatment plan.

During the 1940s, the process was abandoned because of new therapies for seizures. However, approximately 20 to 30% of the epileptic cases failed to reach control of the epileptic seizures. With that failure, the Keto Diet was reintroduced as a management technique.

The Charlie Foundation was founded by the family of Charlie

Abraham in 1994 after his recovery from seizures and other health issues he suffered daily. Charlie, as a youngster, was placed on the diet and continued to use it for five years. As of 2016, he is still functioning successfully without the seizure episodes and is furthering his education as a college student.

The Charlie Foundation appointed a panel of dietitians and neurologists to form an agreement in the form of a statement in 2006. It was written as an approval of the diet, and it stated which cases it would be considered for use. It is noted that the plan is especially recommended for children.

You will be learning the best of two plans when you use the intermittent fasting techniques, specifically the 16/8 plan. Intermittent fasting has grown in popularity in recent years since it has the ability to endorse higher rates of nutrient absorption in the meals you eat.

The plan has also grown in popularity because it doesn't require adherents to change the types of foods radically you are eating or even alter drastically the number of calories you consume in each 24-hour time frame. In fact, the most common type of intermittent fasting is to eat two substantial meals in a day instead of the usual three.

You have so many choices for the intermittent fasting process by using only the ketogenic diet techniques.

This makes the intermittent fasting diet plan an ideal choice for those who find they have difficulty sticking to more strict diet plans, as it only requires changing one habit, which is the number of meals instead of many habits all at once. It's simple enough to manage successfully over a prolonged period while at the same time being efficient enough to provide the type of results that can keep motivation levels high once the novelty of the new way of eating begins to fade.

The secret to intermittent fasting's accomplishment is the simple fact that the body works contrarily in a fasting status versus a fed state, which is when your body actively digests and absorbs food. This process begins some five minutes after you have finished putting food into your body and can last anywhere from three to five hours, depending on how complicated the food is for your body to digest.

While in the fed state, your body is actively producing insulin, which, in turn, makes it harder to burn fat properly. The period after digestion has occurred; the insulin levels start dropping back toward normal. This process can take (in the neighborhood) from 8 to 12 hours, which is the buffer between the fed and fasted state. Once your insulin levels return to normal, the fasted state begins, and this is the period where your body can process fat most effectively. Sadly, many people never reach the point where they can burn fat most efficiently, as they rarely go eight hours, much less twelve hours from some caloric consumption.

These are several celebrities who affirm that the intermittent fasting works.

Nicole Kidman abides the eight-hour fasting rule and sticks with the veggies and proteins as her guidelines for healthier eating. Justin Theroux used intermittent fasting between 7 in the morning until 7 in the evening. It is a bit more of an eating window, but you need to start somewhere. Choose the 16/8 plan and see how it works for you!

CHAPTER 1:

The Keto Diet Plan for Intermittent Fasting

The keto diet will set up your body to deplete the stored glucose. Once that is accomplished, your body will focus on diminishing the stored fat we have saved as fuel. The new technique will begin with 5% for carbs, 75% fats, and 20% for protein daily. Many people don't understand that counting calories don't matter at this point since it is just used as a baseline. Your body doesn't need glucose, which causes these 2 stages:

- *The Stage of Glycogenesis:* The excess of glucose converts itself into glycogen, which is stored in the muscles and liver. Research indicates that only about half of your energy used daily can be saved as glycogen.
- *The Stage of Lipogenesis:* If there is an adequate supply of glycogen in your liver and muscles, any excess is converted to fat and stored.

Your body will have no more food (much like when you are sleeping), making your body burn the fat to create ketones. Once the ketones break down the fats, which generate fatty acids, they will burn-off in the liver through beta-oxidation. Thus, when you no longer have a supply of glycogen or glucose, ketosis begins, and the consumed/stored fat will be used as energy. The Internet provides you with a keto calculator at "keto-calculator.ankerl.com." Begin your process by making a habit of checking your levels when you want to know what essentials your body needs during the course of your dieting plan. You will document your personal information, such as height and weight. The Internet calculator will provide you with essential math.

When the glycerol and fatty acid molecules are released, the ketogenesis process begins, and acetoacetate is produced. The Acetoacetate is converted to two types of ketone units:

- *Acetone:* This is mostly excreted as waste but can also be metabolized into glucose. This is the reason individuals on a ketogenic diet will experience a distinctive smelly breath.

- *Beta-hydroxybutyrate or BHB:* Your muscles will convert the acetoacetate into BHB, which will fuel your brain after you have been on the keto diet for a short time.

You will discover how flexible the ketogenic methods are when coupled with the intermittent fasting techniques. You will lose weight differently with each method, and other people may not have the same goals as you.

For now, as a beginner, you will begin by using the first method, as shown below. This is an important step; you must decide how you want to proceed with your diet plan. It is always best to discuss this essential step with your physician. These are the four methods, for you to understand the different levels of the keto diet plan better:

Keto Method # 1: The standard ketogenic diet (SKD) consists of high-fat, moderate protein, and is low in carbs.

Keto Method # 2: Workout times will call for the targeted keto diet, which is also called TKD. The process consists of adding additional carbohydrates to the diet plan during the times when you are more active.

Keto Method # 3: The cyclical ketogenic diet (CKD) entails a restricted five-day keto diet plan, followed by two high-carbohydrate days.

Keto Method 4: The high-protein keto diet is comparable to the standard keto plan (SKD) in all aspects. You will consume more protein.

Macro Guidelines

Ketogenic 0-20 Carbs Daily: Generally, this low level of carbs is related to a restrictive medical diet, where the patient is restricted to 10 to 15 grams each day to ensure the proper levels of ketosis remains. The Charlie Foundation is one of the plans used to promote the treatment of epilepsy.

Moderate 20-50 Daily Carbs Allowed: If you have diabetes, are obese, or metabolically deranged, this is the plan for you. If you are consuming less than 50 grams daily, your body will achieve a ketosis state, which supplies the ketone bodies.

Liberal 50-100 Daily Carbs Allowed: This option is best if you're active and lean and are attempting to maintain your weight.

Calorie Counting Versus Micros

The short of counting calories is that they don't tell the whole story. You can fill up on the "right" calories, and you may also lose muscle mass. For example, you count one hundred calories of avocado (a fat), which is better than one hundred calories from a cookie (carbs). That is why keto counts the macros (fat, protein, and carbs), not the calories.

Remember This Formula: You will need to calculate your net carbs on some of the recipes you discover on the Internet; some list only the total carbs. If that happens, just take the total carbs listed (-) fiber (=) the total net carb, which is what you need to track an accurate count, so you can remain in ketosis.

Foods Included in the Intermittent Fasting Plan

Fresh Vegetables

You need to add plenty of veggies to your lunch or dinner menu plans. Each of these has the Net Carbs listed per 100 grams or 1/2 cup serving:

- Alfalfa Seeds – Sprouted – 0.2
- Arugula – 2.05

- Asparagus - 6 spears – 2.4
- Hass Avocado – ½ of 1 – 1.8
- Bamboo shoots – 3
- Beans – Green snap – 3.6
- Beet greens – 0.63
- Bell pepper – 2.1
- Broccoli – 4.04
- Cabbage – Savoy – 3
- Carrots – 6.78
- Carrots – baby – 5.34
- Cauliflower – 2.97
- Celery – 1.37
- Chard – 2.14
- Chicory greens – 0.7
- Chives – 1.85
- Coriander – Cilantro leaves – 0.87
- Cucumber with peel – 3.13
- Eggplant – 2.88
- Garlic – 30.96
- Ginger root – 15.77
- Kale – 5.15
- Leeks – bulb (+) lower leaf – 12.35
- Lemongrass – citronella – 25.3
- Lettuce – red leaf – 1.36

- Lettuce – e.g., iceberg – 1.77
- Mushrooms brown – 3.7
- Mustard greens – 1.47
- Onions – yellow – 7.64
- Onions – scallions or spring – 4.74
- Onions – sweet – 6.65
- Peppers – banana – 1.95
- Peppers – red hot chili – 7.31
- Peppers – jalapeno – 3.7
- Peppers – sweet – green – 2.94
- Peppers – sweet – red – 3.93
- Peppers – sweet – yellow – 5.42
- Portabella mushrooms – 2.57
- Pumpkin – 6
- Radishes – 1.8
- Seaweed – kelp – 8.27
- Seaweed – spirulina - 2.02
- Shiitake mushrooms – 4.29
- Spinach – 1.43
- Squash – crookneck – summer – 2.64
- Squash – winter – acorn – 8.92
- Tomatoes – 2.69
- Turnips – 4.63
- Turnip greens – 3.93

- Summer squash - 2.6
- Raw watercress - 3.57
- White mushrooms – 2.26
- Zucchini – 1.5

Chili Peppers: The chemical found in chili peppers is called capsaicin, which will boost your metabolism. The capsaicin will increase the fat and calories you burn during your intermittent fasting plan.

Twenty research studies indicated that you would lose/burn approximately fifty extra calories daily. However, all researchers now agree with the theory. At any rate, enjoy the chili peppers.

Fresh Fruits

It is essential to eat plenty of fruits while on the ketogenic diet plan. Enjoy these according to your daily limits of carbohydrates. This collection of keto fruits are 100 grams each for each 1/2 cup serving:

- Apples – no skin, boiled – 13.6 total carbs
- Apricots – 7.5 total carbs
- Bananas – 23.4 total carbs
- Fresh Blackberries – 5.4 net carbs
- Fresh Blueberries – 8.2 net carbs

- Fresh Strawberries – 3 net carbs
- Cantaloupe – 6 total carbs
- Raw Cranberries – 4 net carbs
- Gooseberries – 8.8 net carbs
- Kiwi – 14.2 total carbs
- Fresh Boysenberries – 8.8 net carbs
- Oranges – 11.7 total carbs
- Peaches – 11.6 total carbs
- Pears – 19.2 total carbs
- Pineapple – 11 total carbs
- Plums – 16.3 total carbs
- Watermelon – 7.1 total carbs

Excellent Spices

Black Pepper: Pepper promotes nutrient absorption in the tissues all over your body, speeds up your metabolism, and improves digestion. The main ingredient of pepper is <u>alkaloid piperine,</u> which gives it the pungent taste. It can boost fat metabolism by as much as 8% for up to several hours after it has been ingested.

Basil: (1 whole leaf, 0.5 gram is <u>0 net carbs)</u> You can use fresh or dried basil to maximize its benefits. Its dark green color is an indication that it also maintains an outstanding source of

magnesium, calcium, and vitamin K, which are excellent for your bones. It also helps with allergies, arthritis, or inflammatory bowel
conditions.

Cinnamon: (1 tsp. is 0.6 grams net carbs) Use cinnamon as part of your daily plan to improve your insulin receptor activity. Just put one-half of a teaspoon of cinnamon into a smoothie, shake, or any other dessert.

Raw Ginger Root is *0.9 net carbs for 1 tbsp and involves* over 25 antioxidants. It maintains hefty anti-inflammatory elements to help reduce muscle aches and the pain and swelling of arthritis. Ginger is best known for its ability to reduce nausea and vomiting and its soothing remedy for sore throats from outbreaks of flu and colds. Have a tea made with hot water simmered with a small amount of lemon and honey and a few slices of ginger as a soothing tonic when you're sick.

Cumin Powder: (1 tbsp. is 2 grams net carbs) Cumin maintains abundant antioxidants which are excellent for your digestion and so much more. It also stimulates the pancreas and gallbladder to secrete bile and enzymes which work to break down the food into usable nutrients your body needs to function healthily. Cumin also helps detoxify the body and is beneficial for several respiratory disorders, including bronchitis and asthma. Cumin is also an excellent source of vitamin A & C, as well as iron, which are all excellent for your immune system.

Cloves: Cloves possess a spicy and sweet flavor, but they also contain powerful natural medicine, including strong antiseptic and germicidal components that can help ward off arthritis pain, gum and tooth pain, and infections. They also relieve digestive problems.

Acceptable Sweeteners

Swerve Granular Sweetener is an excellent choice as a blend. It's made from non-digestible carbs sourced from starchy root veggies and select fruits. Start with 3/4 of a teaspoon for every one teaspoon of sugar. Increase the portion to your taste.

Stevia Drops offer delicious flavors, including hazelnut, vanilla, English toffee, and chocolate. Some individuals think the drops are too bitter, so use only three drops at first to equal one teaspoon of sugar.

Xylitol is at the top of the sugar alternatives, which is an excellent choice to sweeten your teriyaki and barbecue sauce. Its naturally occurring sugar alcohol has a glycemic index (GI) standing of 13.

Beverage Options

Coffee: Your caffeine levels can help increase the metabolic rate by approximately 11%. Studies have shown consumption of a minimum of 270 mg of caffeine—about three cups of coffee—will burn away an additional 100 calories daily. The rates can surely boost your intermittent fasting, as long as you leave it sugar-free.

Tea: Tea is offered as a good source of beverage because of the catechins in the tea conglomerate with the caffeine to help speed up your metabolism. The catechins are an antioxidant and a type of natural phenol which is from the chemical family of flavonoids.

An additional 100 calories can be burned daily to increase your metabolism by four to ten percent with the use of green and oolong tea. The effects may be different with each fasting participant.

Include Healthy Fats & Oils

Extra-Virgin Olive Oil (EVOO): Olive oil dates back to centuries, back when oil was used for anointing kings and priests.

High-quality oil with its low acidity makes the oil have a smoke point as high as 410° Fahrenheit. That's higher than most cooking applications call for, making olive oil more heat-stable than many other cooking fats. It contains (2 tsp.) -0- carbs.

Monounsaturated fats, such as the ones in olive oil, are also linked with better blood sugar regulation, including lower fasting glucose, as well as reducing inflammation throughout the body.

Olive oil also helps prevent cardiovascular disease by protecting the integrity of your vascular system and lowering LDL, which is also called the "bad" cholesterol.

Coconut Oil: You vamp up the fat intake with this high flash-point oil. Enjoy a coconut oil smoothie before your workouts.

Use it with your meats, chicken, fish, or on top of veggies. It will quickly transfer from solid form to oil according to its temperature.

Other Monounsaturated & Saturated Fats

Include these items (listed in grams):

- Avocado, Sesame, Olive, & Flaxseed Oil – 1 tbsp. – 0– net carbs
- Olives – 3 jumbo – 5 large or 10 small – 1 net carb
- Chicken fat, Beef tallow & Duck fat – 1 tbsp. – 0 net carbs
- Unsweetened flaked coconut – 3 tbsp. – 2 net carbs
- Ghee & Unsalted Butter – 1 tbsp. – 0 net carbs
- Egg yolks – 1 large – 0.6 net carbs
- Organic Red Palm oil – e.g., Nutiva - 1 tbsp. – 0 – net carbs
- Various Dressings
- Keto-Friendly Mayonnaise

Other Choices for the Ketogenic Plan

- *Grass-Fed Butter:* You can promote fat loss with butter that is almost carb-free. The butter is a naturally occurring fatty acid which is rich in conjugated linoleic acid (CLA). It is suitable for maintaining weight loss and retaining lean muscle mass.

- *Ghee* is also a great staple for your keto stock, which is also called clarified butter.

- *Yogurt:* Coconut milk is easily digested and contains fats, including lauric acid. Yogurt provides transient bacteria since it feeds existing healthy gut bacteria as they pass through your intestinal tract.

Include These Cold Items

- Full-fat sour cream
- Goat cheese
- Full-fat cream cheese
- Parmesan cheese
- Hard & soft cheeses, e.g., mozzarella or sharp cheddar

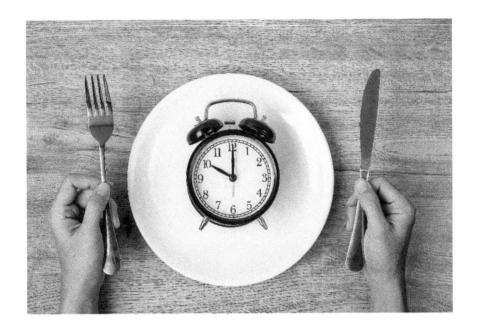

CHAPTER 2:

How to Get Started on the 16/8 Plan

Y ou will still be able to enjoy your regular meals, except you are eating in the eight-hour window.

How to Begin

Step 1: Choose a non-stressful week to begin the ketogenic diet plan.

Step 2: Purge the pantry and fridge.

Step 3: Restock the fridge and pantry with ketogenic food items.

Step 4: Consider skipping one meal each day. Maybe sleep a little longer and have brunch.

Step 5: Initially, don't exceed your net carbs and don't limit the fat and protein you consume.

Step 6: Make a routine. Drink a large glass of water and have a supplement of a ½ teaspoon of MCT oil or 2 teaspoons of coconut oil.

Step 7: Keep track of your ketone levels.

Once you have set your goals and calculated how many carbs you are allowed in one day, it is time to explore the Lean-Gains Method fully.

The 16/8 Method is also called the Lean-Gains Method. The plan is used as a routine targeted explicitly for the removal of body fat and to improve lean muscle mass. One of the most noteworthy benefits of this type of fasting is that it's incredibly flexible so that it will work well if you have a varied schedule. This safe program provides a fasting window of 16 hours, with hours of eating at 8 hours. The easiest way to attempt this schedule is to stop eating after dinner in the evening and wait 14 hours, which means skipping breakfast and picking things up in the early afternoon. For women, you'll fast for 14 hours compared to 16 hours for men before allowing a reasonable quantity of calories for the remaining 8 to 10 hours. Most people find it helpful to either eat two large meals during the 8 or 10-hour feeding period or split that time into three smaller meals since that is the way most people are already programmed.

A study was performed by the Obesity Society, stating that if you have your dinner before 2:00 p.m., your hunger yearnings will be reduced for the remainder of the day. At the same time, your fat-burning reserves are boosted. During the fasting period, you should only consume food items that have zero calories, including black coffee (a splash of cream is excellent), water, diet soda, and sugar-free gum.

Avoid These Food Items

- *Processed Meats:* While protein is an undeniably important part of a healthy diet, seeking your protein from meats, which have been treated, will overload your body full of chemicals. The processed meats tend to be lower in protein while higher in sodium and contain preservatives that can cause a variety of health risks, including asthma and heart disease. Choose from the quality cuts of meat found in most grocery stores.

- *White Flour:* Much like processed meats, by the time white flour has completed the processing, it's utterly devoid of any nutritional value. According to *Care2*, white flour, when consumed as part of a regular diet, has been shown to increase a woman's chance of breast cancer by a shocking 200%.

- *Non-Organic Milk:* Despite being touted as part of a balanced diet, non-organic milk is routinely found to be full of growth hormones. The growth hormones leave behind antibiotics, which, in turn, makes it more difficult for the human body to counter infections, causing an increased chance of colon cancer, prostate cancer, and breast cancer.

- *Farm-Raised Salmon:* Much like processed meat, farm-raised salmons are the least healthy type of an otherwise healthy meal choice. When salmons are raised in close proximity to one another for a prolonged period, they lose much of their natural vitamin D while picking up traces of PCB, DDT, carcinogens, and bromine.

- *Non-Organic Potatoes:* While the starch and carbohydrates it contains are a vital part of a balanced meal, non-organic potatoes are not worth the trouble. They are treated with chemicals while still in the ground, before being treated again; they are sent to the store as "fresh" as possible. These chemicals have been shown to increase the risk of things like birth defects, autism, asthma, learning disabilities, Parkinson's, and

Alzheimer's disease, as well as multiple types of cancer.

Now that you have a good idea of how to proceed with your new way of eating, it is time to review all of the recipes.

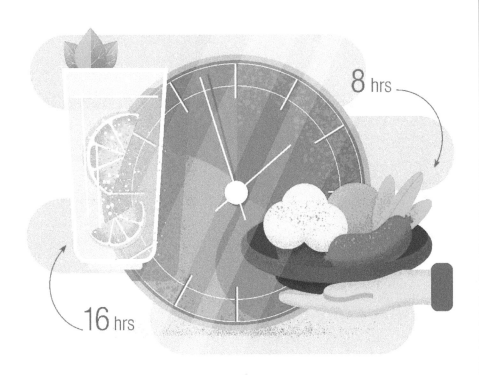

8 hrs

16 hrs

CHAPTER 3:

Breakfast Favorites

1. *Corned Beef & Radish Hash*

Serving Yields Provided: 4

Macro Counts - Each Serving - 0.5 cup each:

- Net Carbs: 1.5 g
- Total Fats: 16 g
- Protein: 23 g
- Calories: 252

Ingredients Needed:

- Olive oil (1 tbsp.)
- Diced onions (.25 cup)
- Radishes (1 cup)
- Kosher salt (.5 tsp.)
- Garlic powder (.25 tsp.)
- Black pepper (.25 tsp.)
- Dried oregano (.5 tsp.)
- Corned beef (12 oz. can) or Finely chopped, packed corned beef (1 cup)

Directions for Preparation:

1. Dice the radishes to .5-inch cuts.

2. Warm the oil in a large sauté pan. Toss in the onions, radishes, salt, and pepper.

3. Sauté the onions and radishes on medium heat until softened (5 min.).

4. Add the oregano, garlic powder, and corned beef to the pan and stir well until combined.

5. Cook using low to medium heat, occasionally stirring for 10 minutes or until the radishes are soft and starting to brown.

6. Press the mixture into the bottom of the pan and cook on high heat for 2 to 3 minutes or until the bottom is crisp and brown.

7. Serve hot.

2. *Creamy Basil Baked Sausage*

Serving Yields Provided: 12

Macro Counts - Each Serving:

- Net Carbs: 4 g
- Total Fats: 23 g
- Protein: 23 g
- Calories: 316

Ingredients Needed:

- Italian sausage, pork, turkey, or chicken (3 lb.)
- Cream cheese (8 oz.)
- Heavy cream (.25 cup)
- Basil pesto (.25 cup)
- Mozzarella (8 oz.)

Directions for Preparation:

1. Warm up the oven to reach 400° Fahrenheit.
2. Lightly spritz a casserole dish with cooking oil spray. Add the sausage to the dish and bake for 30 minutes.
3. Combine the heavy cream, pesto, and cream cheese.
4. Once the sauce is done, pour it over the casserole. Top it off with the cheese.

5. Bake for another 10 minutes. The sausage should reach 160° Fahrenheit in the center when checked with a meat thermometer.

6. *Option 2*: You can also broil for 3 minutes to brown the cheesy layer.

3. *Eggs & Sausage Breakfast Sandwich*

Serving Yields Provided: 1

Macro Counts - Each Serving:

- Net Carbs: 6 g
- Protein: 32g
- Total Fats: 8 g
- Calories: 880

Ingredients Needed:

- Butter (1 tbsp.)
- Large eggs (2)
- Mayonnaise (1 tbsp.)
- Sausage patties, cooked (2)
- Sharp cheddar cheese (2 slices)
- Avocado (2-3 slices)

Directions for Preparation:

1. Warm and melt the butter in a large skillet using the medium heat setting. Place lightly oiled Mason jar rings or silicone egg molds into the pan.
2. Crack the eggs into the rings and use a fork to break the yolks. Gently whisk.

3. Place a lid on the pot and cook for 3 to 4 minutes or until eggs are cooked through. Remove the eggs from the rings.

4. Place one of the eggs on a plate and top it with half of the mayonnaise. Top the eggs with one of the sausage patties, a slice of cheese, and the avocado.

5. Put the second sausage patty on top of the avocado, and top it with the remaining cheese. Spread the remaining mayonnaise on the second cooked egg, and put it on top of the cheese. Serve.

4. *Green Buttered Eggs*

Serving Yields Provided: 2

Macro Counts - Each Serving:

- Net Carbs: 2.5 g
- Total Fats: 27.5 g
- Protein: 12.8 g
- Calories: 311

Ingredients Needed:

- Coconut oil (1 tbsp.)
- Organic butter (2 tbsp.)
- Cloves of garlic (2)
- Fresh cilantro (.5 cup)
- Fresh parsley (.5 cup)
- Fresh thyme leaves (1 tsp.)
- Organic eggs (4)
- Ground cayenne (.25 tsp.)
- Sea salt (.25 tsp.)
- Ground cumin (.25 tsp.)

Directions for Preparation:

1. Mince the garlic, and finely chop the parsley and cilantro.

2. Heat a skillet, melting the oil and butter. Toss in the garlic and sauté about 3 minutes (low setting). Add the thyme. Sauté for another 30 seconds.

3. Toss in the cilantro and parsley using the medium heat setting about three more minutes.

4. Break in the eggs (don't break the yolk).

5. Cover and cook about four to 6 minutes until the yolks are set (runny yolk cooks in 3 to 4 minutes).

6. Serve right away and enjoy.

5. *Keto Hot Cross Buns*

Serving Yields Provided: 8

Macro Counts - Each Serving:

- Net Carbs: 2.1 g
- Total Fats: 3.1 g
- Protein: 5.6 g
- Calories: 84

Ingredients Needed:

- Coconut flour (.33 cup)
- Psyllium husks (.33 cup)
- Baking powder (1 tsp.)
- Swerve granulated sweetener (2 tbsp. or more to taste)
- Salt (.5 tsp.)
- Pumpkin spice (.5 tsp.)
- Cinnamon (.5 tsp.)
- Ground cloves (.5 tsp.)
- Eggs (4 medium)
- Boiling water (1 cup
- Raisins/cacao nibs/chocolate chips
- Powdered sweetener icing mix

Directions for Preparation:

1. Mix each of the dry fixings in a mixing bowl.

2. Whisk and fold in the eggs.

3. Pour in the boiling water and mix until evenly combined.

4. Roll into eight equal balls. Add to a baking pan.

5. Bake in a fan-assisted oven at 350° Fahrenheit for 20–30 minutes.

6. Make the icing. Mark each hot cross bun with a cross using a keto-friendly powdered sweetener confectioners/icing mix and water paste mixture.

6. *Lavender Biscuits*

Serving Yields Provided: 6

Macro Counts - Each Serving:
- Net Carbs: 4 g
- Total Fats: 25 g
- Protein: 10 g
- Calories: 270

Ingredients Needed:
- Coconut oil (.33 cup)
- Almond flour (1.5 cups)
- Egg whites (4)
- Kosher salt (1 pinch)
- Baking powder (1 tsp.)
- Culinary grade lavender buds (1 tbsp.)
- Liquid stevia (4 drops)

Directions for Preparation:
1. Warm up the oven until it reaches 350° Fahrenheit.
2. Spritz a baking sheet with a little coconut oil.
3. Combine the almond flour and coconut oil in a mixing container until it's pea-sized pieces. Set the bowl aside in the fridge.

4. Whisk the eggs until they start foaming. Toss in the salt, lavender, and baking powder. Stir well and mix in the eggs. Mix in with the almond mixture, stirring well.

5. Place the biscuits onto the baking sheet using an ice cream scoop or tablespoon. Pat them, so they become round like a pancake.

6. Bake for 20 minutes and serve.

7. *Pesto Scrambled Eggs*

Serving Yields Provided: 1

Macro Counts - Each Serving:

- Net Carbs: 2.6 g
- Total Fats: 41.5 g
- Protein: 20.4 g
- Calories: 467

Ingredients Needed:

- Eggs (3 large)
- Pesto, green or red (1 tbsp.)
- Butter/Ghee (1 tbsp.)
- Creamed coconut milk/soured cream/crème Fraiche (2 tbsp.)
- Freshly ground black pepper & Himalayan salt (as desired)

Directions for Preparation:

1. Whisk the eggs. Sprinkle with pepper and salt to your liking.
2. Prepare a pan with the butter and wait for it to melt.
3. Combine and prepare the fixings using the low heat setting. Stir well and add the pesto.

4. Take the skillet off of the burner and blend in the crème Fraiche.

5. Combine well. Serve any way you choose.

8. *Porridge*

Serving Yields Provided: 1

Macro Counts - Each Serving:

- Net Carbs: 5.4 g
- Total Fats: 22.8 g
- Protein: 10.1 g
- Calories: 401

Ingredients Needed:

- Salt (1 pinch)
- Coconut cream (4 tbsp.)
- Psyllium husk powder (1 pinch ground)
- Coconut flour (1 tbsp.)
- Flaxseed Egg (1)
- Coconut butter (1 oz.)

Directions for Preparation:

1. Add all of the fixings into a pan, and place it on the stovetop using the low heat setting.

2. Stir continuously to encourage the porridge to thicken. Continue stirring until your preferred thickness is reached.

3. A small amount of coconut milk or a few berries (fresh or frozen) can also be added, to taste.

9. *Pulled Pork Hash*

Serving Yields Provided: 2

Macro Counts - Each Serving:

- Net Carbs: 8 g
- Total Fats: 22 g
- Protein: 21 g
- Calories: 354

Ingredients Needed:

- Lard or fat of choice (2 tbsp.)
- Turnip (1)
- Paprika (.5 tsp.)
- Garlic powder (.25 tsp.)
- Black pepper & salt (.25 tsp. each)
- Brussels sprouts (3)
- Lacinato kale (about 2 leaves, 1 cup)
- Red onion (2 tbsp.)
- Pulled pork (3 oz.)
- Eggs (2)
- *Also Needed*: Large cast-iron skillet

Directions for Preparation:

1. Dice the turnip and slice the Brussel sprouts into halves. Chop the kale and dice the onion.

2. Warm up the oil in a skillet using a medium-high temperature setting. Add the diced turnip and the spices.

3. Cook for approximately 5 minutes.

4. Stir in the rest of the vegetables and cook for another two to 3 minutes until they start to soften.

5. Add in the pork and cook for two more minutes.

6. Make two divots in the hash and crack in the eggs.

7. Cover and cook for 3 to 5 minutes just until the whites are set.

10.   *Pumpkin Pancakes*

Serving Yields Provided: 1

Macro Counts - Each Serving:

- Net Carbs: 4 g
- Total Fats: 56 g
- Protein: 9 g
- Calories: 551

Ingredients Needed:

- Coconut oil (2 tbsp.)
- Eggs (2)
- Cinnamon (.25 tsp.)
- Vanilla extract (.25 tsp.)
- Pumpkin puree (.25 cup)
- Coconut flour (2 tbsp.)
- Butter (2 tbsp.)

Directions for Preparation:

1. Whisk the eggs and puree with the cinnamon and vanilla extract.
2. Slowly, add the coconut flour, whisking until the lumps are gone.
3. Warm up the oil using the medium heat setting.

4. Once the pan is hot, prepare the pancakes until it starts to bubble.

5. Turn it over. Cook until golden brown. Serve with the butter.

11. *Sage & Sausage Patties*

Serving Yields Provided: 8

Macro Counts - Each Serving:
- Net Carbs: 1.4 g
- Total Fats: 11 g
- Protein: 21 g
- Calories: 187

Ingredients Needed:
- Maple extract (1 tsp.)
- Granular swerve sweetener (2 tbsp.)
- Garlic powder (.25 tsp.)
- Pepper (.5 tsp.)
- Cayenne (.125 tsp.)
- Salt (1 tsp.)
- Freshly chopped sage (2 tbsp.)
- Ground pork (1 lb.)
- *For the Pan*: Olive oil (1 tsp.)

Directions for Preparation:
1. Whisk each of the fixings in a mixing container and add the pork. Mix well.
2. Shape the patties to approximately a 1-inch thickness.

3. Add the olive oil or some of the butter to a pan on the stovetop using the medium heat setting. Cook each side for 3 to 4 minutes.

12.   *Smoothie in a Bowl*

Serving Yields Provided: 1

Macro Counts - Each Serving:

- Net Carbs: 4 g
- Total Fats: 35 g
- Protein: 35 g
- Calories: 570

Ingredients Needed:

- Almond milk (.5 cup)
- Spinach (1 cup)
- Heavy cream (2 tbsp.)
- Low-carb protein powder (1 scoop)
- Coconut oil (1 tbsp.)
- Ice (2 cubes)

Ingredients Needed - The Toppings:

- Walnuts (4)
- Raspberries (4)
- Chia seeds 1 tsp.)
- Shredded coconut (1 tbsp.)

Directions for Preparation:

1. Add a cup of spinach to your high-speed blender. Pour in the cream, almond milk, ice, and coconut oil.

2. Blend for a few seconds until it has an even consistency, and all ingredients are combined well. Empty the goodies into a serving dish.

3. Arrange your toppings or give them a toss and mix them together. Of course, you can make it pretty by alternating the strips of toppings.

13.   *Spinach Quiche*

Serving Yields Provided: 6

Macro Counts - Each Serving:

- Net Carbs: 0 g
- Total Fats: 23 g
- Protein: 19g
- Calories: 299

Ingredients Needed:

- Chopped onion (1)
- Olive oil (1 tbsp.)
- Frozen & thawed spinach (10 oz. pkg.)
- Shredded Muenster cheese (3 cups)
- Organic eggs, whisked (5)
- *To Taste*: Black pepper and salt
- *Also Needed*: 9-inch pie plate

Directions for Preparation:

1. Warm the oven in advance to reach 350° Fahrenheit. Lightly grease the dish.
2. Use the medium heat setting to warm a skillet with the oil.

3. Toss in the onions and saute for 4 to 5 minutes. Raise the heat setting to medium-high.

4. Fold in the spinach. Sauté for about two to 3 minutes or until the liquid is absorbed. Cool slightly.

5. Combine the rest of the fixings in a large mixing container and toss with the cooled spinach. Dump into the prepared dish and bake for 30 minutes.

6. Take the quiche out of the oven and cool for at least 10 minutes.

7. Slice into six wedges.

14.   _Tomato Pesto Mug Cake_

Serving Yields Provided: 1

Macro Counts - Each Serving:

- Net Carbs: 4 g
- Total Fats: 45 g
- Protein: 13 g
- Calories: 460

Ingredients Needed:

- Large egg (1)
- Almond flour (2 tbsp.)
- Butter (2 tbsp.)
- Baking powder (.5 tsp.)

Ingredients Needed - The Pesto:

- Almond flour (1 tbsp.)
- Sun-dried tomato pesto (5 tsp.)
- Salt (1 pinch)

Directions for Preparation:

1. Combine each of the fixings in a mug, but keep a little pesto for the garnish.
2. Microwave the cup for 70–80 seconds.

3. Lightly tap the mug on a serving dish. It will fall right out.

4. Top the cake with the pesto and serve.

CHAPTER 4:

Lunchtime Options

15.   *Healthy Thai Pork Salad*

Serving Yields Provided: 2

Macro Counts - Each Serving:

- Net Carbs: 5.2 g
- Total Fats: 33 g
- Protein: 29 g
- Calories: 461

Ingredients Needed - The Sauce:

- Juice & zest of lime (1 lime)
- Chopped cilantro (2 tbsp.)
- Tomato paste (2 tbsp.)
- Soy sauce (2 tbsp. + 2 tsp.)
- Red curry paste (1 tsp.)
- Five Spice (1 tsp.)
- Fish sauce (1 tsp.)
- Red pepper flakes (.25 tsp.)
- Rice wine vinegar (1 tbsp. + 1 tsp.)

- Mango extract (.5 tsp.)
- Liquid stevia (10 drops)

Ingredients Needed - The Salad:

- Romaine lettuce (2 cups)
- Pulled pork (10 oz.)
- Medium chopped red bell pepper (.25 of 1)
- Chopped cilantro (.25 cup)

Directions for Preparation:

1. Zest half of the lime, and chop the cilantro.
2. Mix all of the sauce fixings.
3. Blend the barbecue sauce components and set aside.
4. Pull the pork apart, and make the salad. Pour glaze over the pork with a bit of the sauce.

16.   *Jalapeno Popper Chicken Salad*

Serving Yields Provided: 4

Macro Counts - Each Serving:

- Net Carbs: 0 g
- Total Fats: 38.7 g
- Protein: 46.6 g
- Calories: 532

Ingredients Needed:

- Chicken breast (1.5 lb.)
- Bacon (8 slices, 8 oz.)
- Jalapeños (3)
- Chopped green onion (.5 cup)
- Sour cream or dairy-free mayonnaise (.5 cup)
- Hot sauce (2 tbsp.)
- Garlic powder (.5 tsp.)
- Black pepper (.5 tsp.)
- Salt (.5 tsp.)

Directions for Preparation:

1. Warm the oven to reach 450° Fahrenheit.
2. Prepare a baking sheet with a layer of parchment baking paper.

3. Place raw chicken breast on top of the paper, and place the baking sheet to the oven. Cook until the internal temperature reaches 165° Fahrenheit or about 15 to 18 minutes. Transfer to a large platter and chill slightly.

4. Reduce the oven temperature setting to 425° Fahrenheit.

5. Bake the bacon in the oven until it's crispy (15-20 min.). Transfer to a paper towel-lined plated to remove excess grease. Set aside.

6. Turn on the oven broiler, and prepare a baking tin with paper. Put the jalapeños atop the paper and broil until lightly charred (3 min.). Remove the jalapeños from the oven. Cool slightly before roughly chopping. De-seed jalapeños based on your spice preferences. Transfer the jalapeños to a large mixing bowl.

7. Remove the cooked chicken from the fridge and cube. Crumble the cooked bacon. Transfer both to the mixing bowl of chopped jalapeños.

8. Toss in the rest of the fixings and mix until well-combined.

9. Cover the bowl with a top or foil, and transfer it to the refrigerator to chill for 1 hour before serving.

17. *Jar Salad With Tempeh – Vegan*

Serving Yields Provided: 1

Macro Counts - Each Serving:

- Net Carbs: 4 g
- Protein: 8.1 g
- Total Fats: 18.7 g
- Calories: 215

Ingredients Needed:

- Black pepper & salt (as desired)
- Keto-friendly mayonnaise (4 tbsp.)
- Scallion (.5)
- Cucumber (.25 oz.)
- Red bell pepper (.25 oz.)
- Cherry tomatoes (.25 oz.)
- Leafy greens (.25 oz.)
- Seasoned tempeh (4 oz.)

Directions for Preparation:

1. Chop or shred the vegetables as desired. Layer in the dark leafy greens first, followed by the onions, tomatoes, bell peppers, avocado, and shredded carrot.

2. Top the veggies off with the tempeh or use the same amount of another high-protein option to mix things up in later weeks.

3. Top with keto-vegan mayonnaise before serving.

18.   *Kale Salad*

Serving Yields Provided: 4

Macro Counts - Each Serving:

- Net Carbs: 3 g
- Total Fats: 6 g
- Protein: 4 g
- Calories: 80

Ingredients Needed:

- Salt (.5 tsp.)
- Olive oil (1 tbsp.)
- Kale (1 bunch)
- Lemon juice (1 tbsp.)
- Parmesan cheese (.33 cup)

Directions for Preparation:

1. Use a sharp knife to discard the ribs from the kale and slice into ¼-inch strips.
2. Combine with the salt and oil and toss for about 3 minutes until softened.
3. Toss the cheese, juice, and kale. Serve.

19.   *Simple Red Cabbage Salad*

Serving Yields Provided: 4

Macro Counts - Each Serving:

- Net Carbs: 0.2 g
- Protein: 3 g
- Total Fats: 3 g
- Calories: 131

Ingredients Needed:

- Shredded red cabbage (2 cups)
- Pepper and salt (as desired)
- Coconut sugar (.5 tsp.)
- Red wine vinegar (2 tsp.)
- Coconut oil (1 tbsp.)
- Chopped onion (.25 cup)

Directions for Preparation:

1. Place the steamer basket in the Kitchen robot and add the red cabbage. Lock the top. Set the timer for 1 to 2 minutes. Quick-release the pressure, and remove the basket. Rinse the cabbage under cold water and arrange in four portions.
2. Add the fixings, toss, and serve.

20. *Tuna Salad & Chives*

Serving Yields Provided: 4

Macro Counts - Each Serving:

- Net Carbs: 1 g
- Total Fats: 18 g
- Protein: 20 g
- Calories: 235

Ingredients Needed:

- Tuna in olive oil (15 oz.)
- Mayonnaise (6 tbsp.)
- Chives (2 tbsp.)
- Pepper (.25 tsp.)
- Salt (to taste)

Directions for Preparation:

1. Drain the tuna and finely chop the chives.
2. Add all of the fixings except the lettuce into a mixing bowl.
3. Toss well.
4. Enjoy as-is or spoon into romaine lettuce leaves.

21.   *Warm Peach Scallops Salad*

Serving Yields Provided: 2

Macro Counts - Each Serving:

- Net Carbs: 7 g
- Total Fats: 8g
- Protein: 48 g
- Calories: 130

Ingredients Needed:

- Coconut oil, for the pan (as needed)
- Small scallops (12)
- Sliced peaches (1 whole)
- Sliced onion (.5 of 1)
- Oil (1 tsp.)
- Lemon juice (1 tsp.)
- Arugula leaves (5 oz.)

Directions for Preparation:

1. Warm up the oil in a skillet and add the scallops. Sauté for about 5 minutes per side.

2. Toss the arugula, onion slices, peaches, juice, and oil well.
3. When ready to serve, add the scallops on top of the mixture.

22.   *Vegetarian Club Salad*

Serving Yields Provided: 3

Macro Counts - Each Serving:

- Net Carbs: 5 g
- Total Fats: 26 g
- Protein: 17 g
- Calories: 330

Ingredients Needed:

- Mayonnaise (2 tbsp.)
- Sour cream (2 tbsp.)
- Garlic powder (.5 tsp.)
- Dried parsley (1 tsp.)
- Onion powder (.5 tsp.)
- Milk (1 tbsp.)
- Dijon mustard (1 tbsp.)
- Large hard-boiled eggs (3)
- Cheddar cheese (4 oz.)
- Cherry tomatoes (.5 cup)
- Diced cucumber (1 cup)
- Torn romaine lettuce (3 cups)

Directions for Preparation:

1. Slice the hard-boiled eggs, and cube the cheese with a knife. Cut the tomatoes into halves, and dice the cucumber. Place the containers to the side for now.

2. Prepare the dressing (dried herbs, mayo, and sour cream) and mix well.

3. Add 1 tablespoon of milk to the mixture—and another if it's too thick.

4. Layer the salad with the vegetables, cheese, and egg slices. Scoop a spoonful of mustard in the center, along with a drizzle of dressing.

5. Toss and enjoy!

6. *Notes:* The nutritional count is based on 2 tbsp of dressing.

Soup Choices

23.   *Chicken 'Zoodle' Soup*

Serving Yields Provided: 2
Macro Counts - Each Serving:
- Net Carbs: 4 g
- Total Fats: 16 g
- Protein: 34 g
- Calories: 310

Ingredients Needed:
- Chicken broth (3 cups)
- Chicken breast (1)
- Avocado oil (2 tbsp.)
- Green onion (1)
- Celery stalk (1)
- Cilantro (.25 cup)
- Salt (to taste)
- Peeled zucchini (1)

Directions for Preparation:

1. Chop or dice the breast of the chicken. Pour the oil into a saucepan and cook the chicken until done. Pour in the broth and simmer. Chop the celery and green onions and toss into the pan. Simmer for 3 to 4 more minutes.

2. Chop the cilantro and prepare the zucchini noodles. Use a spiralizer or potato peeler to make the 'noodles.' Add to the pot.

3. Simmer for a few more minutes and season to your liking.

4. Store the leftovers in a glass container in the fridge for 2 to 3 days.

24. *Creamy Chicken Soup*

Serving Yields Provided: 4

Macro Counts - Each Serving:

- Net Carbs: 2 g
- Total Fats: 25 g
- Protein: 18 g
- Calories: 307

Ingredients Needed:

- Butter (2 tbsp.)
- Large breast of chicken (1–2 cups, shredded)
- Cubed cream cheese (4 oz.)
- Garlic seasoning (2 tbsp.)
- Chicken broth (14.5 oz.)
- Salt (to your liking)
- Heavy cream (.25 cup)

Directions for Preparation:

1. Warm a saucepan and melt the butter using the medium heat setting.
2. Add the shredded chicken and toss. Blend in the cream cheese and seasoning, mixing well.

3. When melted, add the heavy cream and broth.

4. Once boiling, lower the heat and cook slowly for 3 to 4 minutes. Season as desired.

25. No-Cook Chilled Avocado & Mint Soup

Serving Yields Provided: 2

Macro Counts - Each Serving:

- Net Carbs: 4 g
- Total Fats: 26 g
- Protein: 4 g
- Calories: 280

Ingredients Needed:

- Romaine lettuce (2 leaves)
- Ripened avocado (1 medium)
- Coconut milk (1 cup)
- Lime juice (1 tbsp.)
- Fresh mint (20 leaves)
- Salt (to your liking)

Directions for Preparation:

1. Combine all of the fixings into a blender and mix well. (You want it thick but not like a puree.)
2. Chill in the refrigerator for 5 to 10 minutes before serving.

Seafood

26.   _Fish Cakes_

Serving Yields Provided: 6

Macro Counts - Each Serving:
- Net Carbs: 0.6 g
- Protein: 1.1 g
- Total Fats: 6.5 g
- Calories: 69

Ingredients Needed:
- Wild-caught, raw, and white boneless fish (1 lb.)
- Cilantro, leaves & stems (.25 cup)
- Pinch of salt (1 pinch)
- Chili flakes (1 pinch)
- Coconut oil or grass-fed ghee, for frying (1-2 tbsp.)
- Avocado or neutral oil, for greasing your hands (as needed)
- Avocados (2 ripe)
- Lemon (1 juiced)
- Salt (1 pinch)

- Water (2 tbsp.)
- *Optional*: Garlic cloves (1-2)
- *Also Needed*: Blender or small food processor

Directions for Preparation:

1. In a food processor, add the fish, herbs, garlic (if using), salt, chili, and fish. Blitz until everything is combined evenly.

2. Use the medium-high heat setting on the stovetop to warm a skillet. Add the ghee or coconut oil. Swirl the pan to coat.

3. Put some oil in your hands, and roll the fish mixture into 6 patties.

4. Add the cakes to the heated frying pan. Fry on each side until golden brown.

5. While the fish cakes are cooking, add all of the dipping sauce ingredients (starting with the lemon juice) into the blender. Blitz until smooth and creamy.

6. When the fish cakes are cooked, serve warm with dipping sauce. Taste the fish, and add more lemon juice or salt to your liking.

27.   *Lobster Salad*

Serving Yields Provided: 4

Macro Counts - Each Serving:

- Net Carbs: 2 g
- Total Fats: 25 g
- Protein: 18 g
- Calories: 307

Ingredients Needed:

- Melted butter (.25 cup)
- Cooked lobster meat (1 lb.)
- Mayonnaise (.25 cup)
- Black pepper (.125 tsp.)

Directions for Preparation:

1. Chop the lobster into bite-sized pieces.
2. Melt and pour the butter over the meat. Toss to coat, and blend in the mayonnaise, along with the pepper.
3. Chill in a covered dish for a minimum of 10 minutes or chill to your liking.

Other Delicious Lunchtime Choices

28. *Mixed Vegetable Patties – Kitchen robot*

Serving Yields Provided: 4

Macro Counts - Each Serving:

- Net Carbs: 3 g
- Total Fats: 10 g
- Protein: 4 g
- Calories: 220

Ingredients Needed:

- Cauliflower florets (1 cup)
- Frozen vegetables (1 bag, mixed)
- Water (1.5 cups)
- Flax meal (1 cup)
- Olive oil (2 tbsp.)

Directions for Preparation:

1. Fill the Kitchen robot with the water, and add the veggies to the steamer basket. Secure the lid and set the timer for 4 to 5 minutes using the high-pressure setting.
2. Quick-release the pressure and drain.
3. Use a potato masher, stirring in the flax meal. Shape into four patties.
4. Select the sauté function in a clean pot and pour in the oil.
5. Prepare the patties until they are golden brown or for about 3 minutes per side before serving.

29. *Pesto Roasted Cabbage & Mushrooms*

Serving Yields Provided: 2

Macro Counts - Each Serving:

- Net Carbs: 8 g
- Total Fats: 56 g
- Protein: 13 g
- Calories: 576

Ingredients Needed:

- Shredded cabbage (.75 cup)
- Pesto sauce (2 tbsp.)
- Hard cheese, Italian style, grated (.2 tbsp.)
- Feta cheese (.25 cup crumbled)
- Chopped basil (1 tbsp.)
- Chopped white mushrooms (.25 cup)
- Olive oil (2 tbsp.)

Directions for Preparation:

1. Warm up the oven in advance to 375° Fahrenheit.
2. Prepare the mushrooms and cabbage and arrange on a baking tray.

3. Spritz with oil and toss evenly.
4. Scoop some pesto sauce on top and toss again.
5. Add the grated cheese over the top and bake for about 20 minutes.
6. Serve with a portion of crumbled feta and basil.

30.   *Sloppy Joes – Vegan*

Serving Yields Provided: 6

Macro Counts - Each Serving:

- Net Carbs: 8.9 g
- Total Fats: 29.9 g
- Protein: 14.7 g
- Calories: 354

Ingredients Needed:

- Hulled hemp seeds (.5 cup)
- Hulled pumpkin seeds - Pepitas (1 cup)
- Chopped walnuts (1 cup)
- Apple cider vinegar (1 tbsp.)
- Prepared mustard (1 tbsp.)
- Tomato paste (6 oz.)
- Garlic powder (.5 tbsp.)
- Onion powder (1 tsp.)
- Granulated sweetener (1 tbsp.)
- Vegetable broth (2 cups)
- Lettuce wraps, for serving

Directions for Preparation:

1. Combine each of the fixings in a dutch oven or soup pot on medium-low heat.

2. Place the top of the pot. Simmer slowly for about 45 minutes, occasionally stirring until the vegetable broth is completely absorbed.

3. Serve on keto rolls or bread.

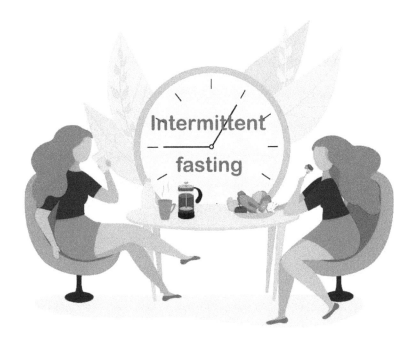

CHAPTER 5:

Tasty Dinner Choices

Poultry

31. *Chicken BBQ Zucchini Boats*

Serving Yields Provided: 4

Macro Counts - Each Serving:

- Net Carbs: 9 g
- Total Fats: 11 g
- Protein: 19 g
- Calories: 212

Ingredients Needed:

- Zucchini (3 halved)
- Boneless skinless chicken breast (1 lb. cooked and shredded)
- BBQ sauce (.5 cup)
- Shredded Mexican cheese (.33 cup)

- Avocado (1 sliced)
- Halved cherry tomatoes (.5 cup)
- Diced green onions (.25 cup)
- Keto-friendly ranch dressing (3 tbsp. to drizzle)
- *Also Needed:* 9x13 casserole dish

Directions for Preparation:

1. Warm up the oven to 350° Fahrenheit.
2. Scoop the seeds out of the zucchini halves, leaving a ½-inch hole carved out of the center (similar to a boat). Place the zucchini flesh side up into the casserole dish.
3. Add shredded chicken and BBQ sauce to a small bowl. Toss to coat all the chicken with the barbeque sauce.
4. Fill the zucchini boats with the BBQ chicken mixture. (about .25 to .33 cup for each zucchini boat)
5. Sprinkle with Mexican cheese on top.
6. Bake for 15 minutes. (Note: If you would like it to be more tender, bake for an additional 5 to 10 minutes to your desired tenderness)
7. Remove from oven.
8. Garnish with avocado, tomatoes, green onion, and a drizzle of ranch dressing. Serve.

32. *Roasted Chicken & Tomatoes*

Serving Yields Provided: 2

Macro Counts - Each Serving:

- Net Carbs: 5 g
- Protein: 16 g
- Total Fats: 16 g
- Calories: 233

Ingredients Needed:

- Olive oil (1 tbsp.)
- Plum tomatoes (2 quartered)
- Chicken legs, bone-in with skin (2)
- Paprika (1 tsp.)
- Ground oregano (1 tsp.)
- Balsamic vinegar (1 tbsp.)

Directions for Preparation:

1. Set the oven temperature setting to 350° Fahrenheit. Grease a roasting pan with a spritz of oil.
2. Rinse and lightly dab the chicken legs dry with a paper towel. Prepare using the oil and vinegar over the skin. Season with paprika and oregano.

3. Arrange the legs in the pan, along with the tomatoes around the edges.
4. Cover with a layer of foil and bake for 1 hour. Baste to prevent the chicken from drying out.
5. Discard the foil and increase the temperature to 425° Fahrenheit.
6. Bake 15 to 30 minutes more until browned and the juices run clear.
7. Serve with a side salad.

33. *Sesame Chicken Egg Roll in a Bowl*

Serving Yields Provided: 8

Macro Counts - Each Serving:

- Net Carbs: 3.3 g
- Protein: 15 g
- Total Fats: 19.5 g
- Calories: 267

Ingredients Needed:

- Toasted sesame oil (3 tbsp.)
- Red onion (1 small, about .5 cup)
- Garlic (4 cloves)minced
- Green onions (5)
- Boneless chicken breast or thigh (1.5 lb.)
- Black pepper (.5 tsp.)
- Sea salt (1 tsp.)
- Ginger powder (1 tsp.)
- Sriracha sauce or garlic chili sauce (1 tbsp. + 1 tsp.)
- Broccoli slaw (20 oz.)
- Unseasoned rice vinegar (2 tbsp.)
- Coconut aminos (.25 cup)
- Toasted sesame seeds (1 tbsp.)

Directions for Preparation:

1. Chop the red onion and slice the onions on the bias (separate the white and green portions). Mince the garlic. Cut the chicken into bite-sized pieces.

2. Warm up the oil in a large pan using the medium-high temperature setting.

3. Toss in the garlic, red onion, and white portion of the green onions into the skillet. Sauté until the onions are translucent and the garlic is fragrant.

4. Add the chicken, salt, pepper, ginger, and Sriracha to the pan. Sauté until it's fully cooked.

5. Add the aminos, broccoli slaw, and vinegar. Sauté until the broccoli is tender.

6. Garnish the dish using the green parts of the onions, and sesame seeds before serving. Add Sriracha sauce as desired.

Pork

34.   *Pan-Fried Chops*

Serving Yields Provided: 3

Macro Counts - Each Serving:

- Net Carbs: 4.2 g
- Total Fats: 27 g
- Protein: 22 g
- Calories: 385

Ingredients Needed:

- Coconut flour (.5 cup)
- Salt and black pepper (1 tsp. each)
- Pork chops (3)
- Butter (1 tbsp.)

Directions for Preparation:

1. Combine all of the dry fixings in a large mixing container.
2. Pat the chops dry with a paper towel.
3. Melt the butter in a skillet on the stovetop.

4. Cover the chops with the mixture and prepare each side for 4 to 5 minutes.

5. Serve with your favorite side dishes.

35.   *Parmesan Crusted Pork Chops*

Serving Yields Provided: 14

Macro Counts - Each Serving:

- Net Carbs: 3 g
- Total Fats: 34 g
- Protein: 33 g
- Calories: 354

Ingredients Needed:

- Parmesan cheese (6 oz.)
- Pork chops (14)
- Large eggs (2)
- Almond flour (.75 cup)
- Pepper and salt (to taste)
- *For Frying:* Bacon grease

Directions for Preparation:

1. Heat the oven to 400° Fahrenheit.
2. Grate the parmesan and mix with the flour and spices.
3. Whisk the eggs in a shallow dish.
4. Dip the chops in the eggs and then the parmesan mixture.

5. Fry on each side using the bacon grease for 1 minute.

6. Arrange on a baking dish in the oven, baking until done. Serve.

36. Slow-Cooked Kalua Pork & Cabbage

Serving Yields Provided: 12

Macro Counts - Each Serving:
- Net Carbs: 4 g
- Total Fats: 13 g
- Protein: 22 g
- Calories: 227

Ingredients Needed:
- Boneless pork shoulder butt (3 lb.)
- Head of cabbage (1 medium, approx. 2 lb.)
- Bacon (7 strips, divided)
- Coarse sea salt (1 tbsp.)
- *Suggested*: 6-quart slow cooker

Directions for Preparation:
1. Coarsely chop the cabbage. Trim the fat from the roast.
2. Layer most of the bacon in the cooker. Dust the salt over the roast and place the rest of the bacon on top. Close the top and cook on low for 8 to 10 hours.

3. At that time, drop in the cabbage and continue cooking, covered for another hour until it's tender (time may vary).

4. When the roast is done, remove, and shred. Use a slotted spoon to arrange the cabbage in the serving dish.

5. Use some of the slow cooker juices on the side for dipping.

37. _Stuffed Pork Tenderloin on the Grill_

Serving Yields Provided: 6

Macro Counts - Each Serving:

- Net Carbs: 3 g
- Total Fats: 6 g
- Protein: 29 g
- Calories: 194

Ingredients Needed:

- Pork tenderloin or venison (2 lb.)
- Feta cheese (.5 cup)
- Gorgonzola cheese (.5 cup)
- Onion (1 tsp.)
- Cloves of garlic (2 cloves)
- Crushed almonds (2 tbsp.)
- Sea Salt & black pepper (.5 tsp. each)

Directions for Preparation:

1. Warm up the grill.
2. Create a pocket in the tenderloin using a sharp knife.
3. Chop the onion and mince the garlic.
4. Combine the cheeses, onions, almonds, and garlic.
5. Stuff the pork pocket and seal using a skewer.

6. Grill until done (approx. 1 hr.) with the lid closed (about 300-350° Fahrenheit).

7. The center of the meat should reach 150° Fahrenheit.

8. Cover it with foil, and let it rest for about 15 minutes before serving.

Fish Seafood Options

38.   *Lemon Shrimp*

Serving Yields Provided: 2

Macro Counts - Each Serving:

- Net Carbs: 2.5 g
- Total Fats: 27 g
- Protein: 22.5 g
- Calories: 335

Ingredients Needed:

- Olive oil (.25 cup)
- Large shrimp (.5 lb.)
- Garlic cloves (3)
- Lemon (1 wedge)
- Pepper and salt (as desired)

Directions for Preparation:

1. Sauté the garlic with the cayenne along with the olive oil using medium heat.
2. Peel the shrimp and cook 2–3 minutes per side.

3. Dust the shrimp with the pepper, salt, and a lemon wedge.

4. Use the remainder of the garlic oil for a dipping sauce.

39. _**Skillet Fried Cod**_

Serving Yields Provided:

Macro Counts - Each Serving: 4

- Net Carbs: 1 g
- Total Fats: 7 g
- Protein: 21 g
- Calories: 160

Ingredients Needed:

- Ghee (3 tbsp.)
- Cod fillets (4, .33 lb. ea.)
- Minced garlic cloves (6)
- _Optional:_ Garlic powder
- _Optional:_ Salt

Directions for Preparation:

1. Melt the ghee, and add half of the garlic into a skillet.
2. Arrange the fillets in the pan using medium-high heat. Sprinkle with garlic, pepper, and salt.
3. Once it turns white halfway up its side, turn it over, and add the remainder of the minced garlic. Continue cooking until it flakes easily.
4. Serve with some ghee/garlic from the pan.

Beef Options

40. *Ground Beef Vegetable Skillet*

Serving Yields Provided:
Macro Counts - Each Serving:
- Net Carbs: g
- Total Fats: g
- Protein: g
- Calories:

Ingredients Needed:
- Extra virgin olive oil (2 tbsp.)
- Grass-fed, extra-lean ground beef (1 lb.)
- Clove of garlic (1)
- Onions (.5 cup)
- Red bell peppers (.5 cup)
- Zucchini (1 medium)
- Asparagus (.5 lb.)
- Dijon mustard (1 tsp.)
- Tomato passata or tomato sauce (.25 cup)
- Dried oregano (.5 tsp.)

- *Optional*: Crushed red pepper (.125 tsp.)
- Salt and freshly ground black pepper (as desired)
- *For the Garnish*:
- Freshly chopped parsley (to your liking)
- Crumbled feta cheese (1 tbsp.)

Directions for Preparation:

1. Mince or dice the garlic, onions, and peppers. Quarter the zucchini, and slice the asparagus into three segments each.
2. Warm up a large skillet using the medium-high heat setting, and add the olive oil
3. Toss in the garlic and beef. Break apart as it cooks. Stir it occasionally and cook for about 7 minutes until it's no longer pink. Remove the meat from the skillet, and set it aside for now.
4. Fold in the onions and red bell peppers. Simmer until the onions are softened or about 3 to 4 minutes. Pour in a little bit of olive oil to help sauté the veggies as needed.
5. Toss in the zucchini and asparagus. Simmer for another 3 to 5 minutes.
6. Return the beef to the skillet, and mix everything together.
7. Simmer for one to two additional minutes.

41.   *Hamburger Stroganoff*

Serving Yields Provided: 1

Macro Counts - Each Serving:

- Net Carbs: 6 g
- Total Fats: 28 g
- Protein: 39 g
- Calories: 447

Ingredients Needed:

- Lean ground beef (1 lb.)
- Sliced mushrooms (8 oz.)
- Minced cloves of garlic (2)
- Butter (2 tbsp.)
- Sour cream (1.25 cups)
- Water or dry white wine (.33 cup)
- Lemon juice (1 tsp.)
- Dried parsley (1 tsp.)
- Paprika (.25 tsp.)
- *Optional*: Freshly chopped parsley (1 tbsp.)

Directions for Preparation:

1. Warm a skillet to sauté the onions and garlic using 1 tbsp butter.

2. Mix the beef into the pan and sprinkle with pepper and salt if desired. Cook until done and set to the side.

3. Add the remainder of the butter, mushrooms, and the wine or water to the pan. Cook until half of the liquid is reduced and the mushrooms are soft.

4. Take it away from the heat, and add the paprika and sour cream.

5. On low heat, stir in the meat and lemon juice. Use additional spices for flavoring if desired.

42. *Mongolian Beef*

Serving Yields Provided: 6

Macro Counts - Each Serving:

- Net Carbs: 1.99 g
- Total Fats: 19 g
- Protein: 37 g
- Calories: 339

Ingredients Needed:

- Flank steak (1.5 lb.)
- *Optional:* Crushed red pepper flakes (.25 tsp.)
- Fish sauce (1 tbsp.)
- Garlic cloves (3)
- Toasted sesame oil (2 tbsp.)
- Gluten-free coconut aminos (2 tbsp.)
- Golden monk fruit sweetener, e.g., Lakanto (.5 cup)
- Avocado oil (1 tbsp.)
- Fresh ginger (1 tbsp.)
- Glucomannan powder or xanthan gum (1.5 tsp.)
- Green onions (2 tbsp.)

Directions for Preparation:

1. Mince the cloves of garlic, and grate the piece of ginger. Thinly slice the onions.

2. Cutting against the grain, slice the steak into thin strips then into one to two-inch pieces. Set aside.

3. Whisk the fish sauce, red pepper flakes, minced garlic, aminos, sesame oil, and monk fruit sweetener.

4. Add the sliced steak and rotate steak strips until all meat is coated in marinade. Cover the bowl and transfer to the fridge to marinate for 30 minutes.

5. Once the steak has finished marinating, heat the avocado oil in a skillet using the medium temperature setting. Add the steak, marinade, and grated ginger to the pan. Cook the steak until browned, flipping as needed. Remove from the burner.

6. Spoon out .5 cup of the sauce from the pan and transfer to a mixing bowl. Sprinkle the glucomannan powder on top of the sauce. Whisk the fixings together until the sauce thickens.

7. Pour the sauce back into the pan.

8. Serve the beef in bowls on its own or atop cauliflower rice, and garnish it with sliced green onions.

9. Consume within 2 to 3 days, or freeze it for 2 months.

43.   *Nacho Skillet Steak*

Serving Yields Provided: 5

Macro Counts - Each Serving:

- Net Carbs: 6 g
- Total Fats: 31 g
- Protein: 19 g
- Calories: 385

Ingredients Needed:

- Butter (1 tbsp.)
- Beef round tip steak (8 oz.)
- Melted refined coconut oil (.33 cup)
- Turmeric (.5 tsp.)
- Chili powder (1 tsp.)
- Cauliflower (1.5 lb.)
- Shredded cheddar cheese (1 oz.)
- Shredded Monterey Jack cheese (1 oz.)

Optional Toppings:

- Canned jalapeno slices (1 oz.)
- Sour cream (.33 cup)
- Avocado (5 oz.)

Directions for Preparation:

1. Set the oven temperature to 400° Fahrenheit.
2. Cut the cauliflower into chip-like shapes.
3. Combine the turmeric, chili powder, and coconut oil in a mixing dish.
4. Toss in the cauliflower, and add it to a baking tin. Set the baking timer for 20 to 25 minutes.
5. Over medium-high heat in a cast iron skillet, add the butter. Cook until both sides of the meat is done, flipping just once. Let it rest for 5–10 minutes. Thinly slice and sprinkle with some pepper and salt.
6. When done, transfer the florets to the skillet, and add the steak strips. Top it with the cheese and bake for 5–10 more minutes.
7. Serve with your favorite garnish, but you have to count those carbs.

44.   *Slow-Cooked London Broil*

Serving Yields Provided: 4

Macro Counts - Each Serving:

- Net Carbs: 2.5 g
- Protein: 47 g
- Total Fats: 18 g
- Calories: 409

Ingredients Needed:

- Minced garlic (2 tsp.)
- London broil (2 lb.)
- Dijon mustard (1 tbsp.)
- Reduced sugar ketchup (2 tbsp.)
- Coconut Aminos/ your choice soy sauce substitute (2 tbsp.)
- Coffee (.5 cup)
- Chicken broth (.5 cup)
- White wine (.25 cup)
- Onion powder (2 tsp.)

Directions for Preparation:

1. Arrange the beef in the cooker. Cover both sides with the mustard, soy sauce, ketchup, and minced garlic.

2. Pour the liquid components into the cooker, and give it a sprinkle of the onion powder.

3. Cook it for 4 to 6 hours.

4. When the timer buzzes, shred the meat. Combine with the juices and serve.

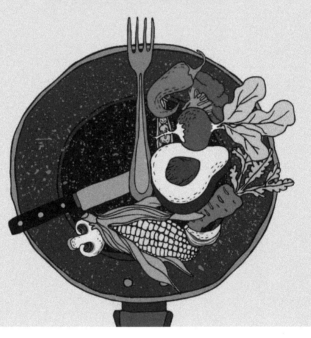

INTERMITTENT FASTING

CHAPTER 6:

Snacktime Treats

45. *Grilled Zucchini & Cheese Sandwich*

Serving Yields Provided: 2

Macro Counts - Each Serving:

- Net Carbs: 6 g
- Total Fats: 90.1 g
- Protein: 29 g
- Calories: 936

Ingredients Needed:

- Shredded zucchini (2 cups)
- Egg (1)
- Shredded Italian-style hard cheese (.125 cup)
- Shredded cheddar cheese (.5 cup)
- Green sliced onions, sliced (.25 cup)
- Cornstarch (.25 tbsp.)
- Coconut oil (4 tbsp.)

Directions for Preparation:

1. Shred the zucchini and wrap in towels for about 1 hour. Use a skillet or other heavy object over it to squeeze out the extra liquids.

2. Combine with the egg, cornstarch, cheese, and onions. Sprinkle with pepper and salt. Toss well.

3. Pour oil in a skillet to cover the pan, and warm it using the medium heat temperature setting. When it's hot, add about ¼ of the zucchini mixture into the skillet, shaping it into a square.

4. Cook it until golden, and drain the grease using paper towels.

5. In the same pan, add two zucchini patties and top with cheddar cheese. Add the second patty on top to make a sandwich.

46.   *Pepper Jack Mug Melt*

Serving Yields Provided: 1

Macro Counts - Each Serving:

- Net Carbs: 3.83 g
- Total Fats: 18 g
- Protein: 22.4g
- Calories: 268

Ingredients Needed:

- Roast beef deli slices (2 oz.)
- Diced green chiles (1.5 tbsp.)
- Sour cream (1 tbsp.)
- Shredded pepper jack cheese (1.5 oz.)

Directions for Preparation:

1. Tear apart the roast beef, and layer it in the bottom of the dish.
2. First, spread half of the sour cream, followed by a ½ tablespoon of the green chili.
3. Layer it with ½ ounce of the pepper cheese. Follow with another layer.
4. Microwave for 1 to 2 minutes until the cheese melts. Serve.

47.   *Smoked Salmon & Cream Cheese Roll-Ups*

Serving Yields Provided: 2

Macro Counts - Each Serving:

- Net Carbs: 3 g
- Total Fats: 22 g
- Protein: 14g
- Calories: 268

Ingredients Needed:

- Chopped scallions, green and white parts (2 tbsp.)
- Dijon mustard (1 tsp.)
- Grated lemon zest (1 tsp.)
- Room temperature cream cheese (4 oz.)
- Cold smoked salmon (12 slices, 4 oz.)
- Salt & Freshly ground black pepper (as desired)

Directions for Preparation:

1. In a blender or food processor, add the lemon zest, cream cheese, scallions, and mustard. Flavor with pepper and salt according to taste. Mix until creamy smooth.

2. Spread the cheese mix on both sides of the salmon and roll. Arrange with the seam side down on a platter.

3. Cover it with plastic and place in the fridge until it's ready to eat. They will remain fresh for about 3 days.

48.   *Spicy Beef Wraps*

Serving Yields Provided: 2

Macro Counts - Each Serving:

- Net Carbs: 4 g
- Total Fats: g
- Protein: 30 g
- Calories: 375

Ingredients Needed:

- Coconut oil (1–2 tbsp.)
- Onion (.25 of 1)
- Ground beef (.66 lb.)
- Chopped cilantro (2 tbsp.)
- Red bell pepper (1)
- Fresh ginger (1 tsp.)
- Cumin (2 tsp.)
- Garlic cloves (4)
- Pepper and salt (as preferred)
- Large cabbage leaves (8)

Directions for Preparation:

1. Dice the bell pepper, onion, ginger, and garlic.
2. Warm a frying pan and pour some oil.

3. Sauté the peppers, onions, and ground beef using medium heat.
4. When done, add the black pepper, salt, cumin, ginger, cilantro, and garlic.
5. Scoop the mixture onto each leaf, fold, and serve.

49. *Steak Pinwheels*

Serving Yields Provided: 6

Macro Counts - Each Serving:

- Net Carbs: 2 g
- Total Fats: 19.5 g
- Protein: 54.5 g
- Calories: 414

Ingredients Needed:

- Flank steak (2 lb.)
- Mozzarella cheese (8 oz. pkg.)
- Spinach (about 1.75 cups, 1 bunch)

Directions for Preparation:

1. Warm the oven to 350° Fahrenheit.
2. Slice the steak into six portions, and remove all of the "hard" fat. Beat it thin with a mallet.
3. Shred the cheese using a food processor and sprinkle the steak. Roll it up and tie with a piece of cooking twine or a skewer.
4. Line the pan with the pinwheels and place on a layer of spinach. Bake until done (25 min.).

50.   *Stuffed Mushrooms*

Serving Yields Provided: 4

Macro Counts - Each Serving:

- Net Carbs: 3 g
- Total Fats: 22 g
- Protein: 5 g
- Calories: 124

Ingredients Needed:

- Portobello mushrooms (4)
- Olive oil (2 tbsp.)
- Blue cheese (1 cup)
- Fresh thyme (1 pinch)
- Salt (as desired)

Directions for Preparation:

1. Warm the oven to 350° Fahrenheit.
2. Cut the stems from the mushrooms and chop them to bits.
3. Mix with the thyme, salt, and crumbled blue cheese and stuff the mushrooms.
4. Spritz with some of the oil.
5. Bake for 15 to 20 minutes. Serve as a delicious snack or side dish.

Sweet Snacks

51. *Peanut Butter Protein Bars*

Serving Yields Provided: 12 bars

Macro Counts - Each Serving:

- Net Carbs: 3 g
- Total Fats: 14 g
- Protein: 7 g
- Calories: 172

Ingredients Needed:

- Keto-friendly chunky peanut butter (1 cup)
- Egg whites (2)
- Almonds (.5 cup)
- Cashews (.5 cup)
- Almond meal (1.5 cups)

Directions for Preparation:

1. Warm up the oven ahead of time to 350° Fahrenheit.
2. Combine all of the fixings and add to the prepared dish.
3. Bake for 15 minutes.

4. Cut into 12 pieces once they're cool.

5. Store in the fridge to keep them fresh.

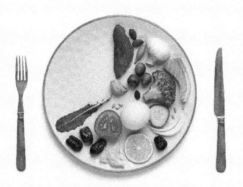

CHAPTER 7:

Dessert Favorites

52.   *No-Bake Cheesecake*

Serving Yields Provided: 6

Macro Counts - Each Serving:

- Net Carbs: 5 g
- Total Fats: 25 g
- Protein: 7 g
- Calories: 247

Ingredients Needed - The Crust:

- Almond flour (2 tbsp.)
- Melted coconut oil (2 tbsp.)
- Swerve Confectioners or equivalent (2 tbsp.)
- Crushed salted almonds (2 tbsp.)

Ingredients Needed - The Filling:

- Gelatin (1 tsp.)
- Swerve confectioners or equivalent (.25 cup)

- Cream cheese (16 oz. pkg.)
- Unsweetened almond milk (.5 cup)
- Vanilla extract (1 tsp.)

Directions for Preparation:

1. Prepare the crust by combining all of the fixings under the crust section. Place one heaping tablespoon into the bottom of the dessert cups. Press the mixture down and set aside.

2. Prepare the filling. Mix the sweetener and gelatin. Pour in the milk and stir (5 min.). Whip the vanilla beans and cream cheese with a mixer using the medium setting until creamy. Add the gelatin mixture slowly until well-incorporated.

3. Pour the mixture over the crust of each cup. Chill for 3 hours, minimum.

53. *No-Bake Chocolate Fudge Haystacks*

Serving Yields Provided: 12

Macro Counts - Each Serving:

- Net Carbs: 1.5 g
- Total Fats: 18 g
- Protein: 2 g
- Calories: 172

Ingredients Needed:

- Softened cream cheese (4 oz.)
- Erythritol sweetener (.75 cup)
- Softened unsalted butter (.5 cup)
- Unsweetened cocoa powder (.25 cup)
- Coarse sea salt (.125 tsp.)
- Unsweetened desiccated/shredded coconut (1 cup)
- Sugar-free vanilla extract (1 tsp.)
- Chopped walnuts (.33 cups)

Directions for Preparation:

1. Blend the cocoa powder, sweetener, cheese, and butter.
2. Stir in the walnuts, coconut, salt, and vanilla extract.

3. Scoop out 1-inch balls to make haystacks. Chill for approximately 30 minutes or longer.

4. Store in the refrigerator or freezer for best results.

54. *Peanut Butter Fudge*

Serving Yields Provided: 20

Macro Counts - Each Serving:

- Net Carbs: 6 g
- Total Fats: 11 g
- Protein: 4 g
- Calories: 135

Ingredients Needed:

- Coconut oil (3 tbsp.)
- Smooth peanut butter, keto-friendly (12 oz.)
- Coconut cream (4 tbsp.)
- Maple syrup (4 tbsp.)
- Salt (1 pinch)

Directions for Preparation:

1. Prepare a baking sheet with a layer of parchment paper.
2. Melt the syrup and coconut oil using the medium heat setting on the stovetop.
3. Stir in the salt, coconut cream, and peanut butter. Pour the mixture into the prepared dish and chill in the fridge for at least 1 hour.
4. Slice into pieces and store or serve.

55. *Pumpkin Caramel Bundt Cake*

Serving Yields Provided: 16

Macro Counts - Each Serving:

- Net Carbs: 5 g
- Total Fats: 16.5 g
- Protein: 8 g
- Calories: 212

Ingredients Needed - The Cake:

- Almond flour (2.5 cups)
- Coconut flour (.5 cup)
- Swerve sweetener (.66 cup)
- Baking powder (1 tbsp.)
- Unflavored whey protein powder (.33 cup)
- Cinnamon (2 tsp.)
- Ginger (1 tsp.)
- Salt (.5 tsp.)
- Cloves (.25 tsp.)
- Pumpkin puree (1.5 cups)
- Large eggs (4)
- Melted butter (.25 cup)
- Water (.5 to .66 cup)
- Vanilla extract (1 tsp.)

Ingredients Needed - The Glaze:

- Butter (.25 cup)
- Molasses for color and flavor (1 tsp.)
- Powdered Swerve sweetener (.5 cup)
- Caramel flavor (.5 tsp.)
- Whipping cream (2 tbsp.)

Directions for Preparation - Cake Preparation:

1. Warm up the oven to 325° Fahrenheit.
2. Grease the pan well. Whisk the coconut flour, almond flour, sweetener, protein powder, salt, baking powder, cloves, and ginger in the mixing bowl.
3. Fold in the eggs, pumpkin puree, 1/2 cup water, butter, and vanilla extract. Add small amounts of water as needed for a thick consistency.
4. Empty the batter into the greased pan.
5. Bake 55 to 60 minutes. Test for doneness.
6. Remove and let cool 15 minutes.
7. Place onto the rack to cool.

Directions for Preparation - The Glaze:

1. In the pan, using low heat, melt butter with molasses or yacon syrup. Stir it until smooth.

2. Take the pan off the burner and stir in powdered sweetener, caramel extract, and whipping cream.

3. Drizzle over the cooled cake. It's also grain-free.

56. *Raspberry Fudge*

Serving Yields Provided: 12

Macro Counts - Each Serving:

- Net Carbs: 4.4 g
- Protein: 2.6 g
- Total Fats: 25.3 g
- Calories: 242

Ingredients Needed:

- Cream cheese (16 oz.)
- Butter (1 cup)
- Heavy cream (2 tbsp.)
- White sugar substitute (.25 cup)
- Unsweetened cocoa powder (6 tbsp.)
- Vanilla extract (2 tsp.)
- Raspberry extract (1 tsp.)
- Chopped walnuts (.33 cup)

Directions for Preparation:

1. Take the cream cheese and butter out of the fridge ahead of time until it is cooled to room temperature.
2. Mix the cream cheese and butter in a mixing bowl with the mixer.

3. When smooth, mix with the rest of the fixings until well-incorporated.

4. Microwave it using the high setting for 30 seconds. Blend it with the mixer again until smooth.

5. Empty the mixture into the prepared pan (1-inch layer). Cover it and chill for at least 2 hours in the fridge.

6. Slice into 12 portions.

7. Serve or store in the fridge.

57.   *Raspberry Ice Cream*

Serving Yields Provided: 5

Macro Counts - Each Serving - .5 cup each::

- Net Carbs: 3 g
- Protein: 1 g
- Total Fats: 16 g
- Calories: 183

Ingredients Needed:

- Heavy cream (or coconut cream (1 cup)
- Frozen raspberries (2 cups)
- Powdered erythritol or any sweetener, to taste (.33 cup)

Directions for Preparation:

1. Pour the cream into a blender. Blend until stiff peaks form (you can also use a hand mixer if your blender isn't powerful enough to whip the cream).
2. Add the frozen raspberries and sweetener to the blender. Puree until incorporated. Adjust the sweetener to taste, and puree it again if needed.

3. *Note:* If you prefer firmer ice cream; you can run the mixture through an ice cream maker, or place it in the freezer to firm up.

4. If you're using the freezer, stir every 30–60 minutes for the first couple hours to break up any ice crystals.

58.   *Sugar-Free Fudgesicles*

Serving Yields Provided: 8

Macro Counts - Each Serving:

- Net Carbs: 1.6 g
- Protein: 1.44 g
- Total Fats: 11.2 g
- Calories: 118

Ingredients Needed:

- Heavy cream (1 cup)
- Almond or cashew milk unsweetened (1 cup)
- Unsweetened cocoa powder (.33 cup)
- Swerve Sweetener (.33 cup)
- Vanilla extract or peppermint extract (1 tsp.)
- Xanthan gum (.25 tsp.)
- *Also Needed:* Wooden sticks

Directions for Preparation:

1. Whisk the swerve, cream, milk, and cocoa powder in a saucepan using the medium-high heat setting. Cook for 1 minute after it starts to boil.
2. Transfer the pan from the burner, and add the flavoring.
3. Add the xanthan gum and whisk well.

4. Chill for a minimum of 10 minutes before pouring into the molds.

5. Freeze for at least another hour. Push the popsicle sticks into the mixture, but not all the way, and then return the mold to the freezer.

6. When you're ready to enjoy it, pour a bit of hot water over the mold to release the popsicles.

59. _Vanilla Shortbread Cookies_

Serving Yields Provided: 16

Macro Counts - Each Serving:

- Net Carbs: 1 g
- Total Fats: 12 g
- Protein: 3 g
- Calories: 126

Ingredients Needed:

- Almond flour (2 cups)
- Erythritol (.33 cup)
- Salt (1 pinch)
- Egg (1 large)
- Softened unsalted butter (.5 cup)
- Vanilla extract (1 tsp.)

Directions for Preparation:

1. Warm the oven to reach 300° Fahrenheit.
2. Combine the almond flour with the salt, erythritol, salt, and vanilla extract.
3. Toss in the butter and rub into the dry ingredients until fully mixed.
4. Fold in the whisked egg.

5. Roll tablespoon-sized pieces of the mixture into balls.

6. Press onto a lined cookie sheet. Leave a gap between the cookies.

7. Bake until the edges are browned (for 15 to 25 min.).

8. The cookies will firm up as they cool. Leave to cool before storing in an airtight jar.

9. *Note*: It's recommended to use gloves to prevent the mixture from sticking to your hands.

60.   *Vanilla Sour Cream Cupcake*

Serving Yields Provided: 12

Macro Counts - Each Serving:

- Net Carbs: 2 g
- Protein: 4 g
- Total Fats: 11 g
- Calories: 128

Ingredients Needed:

- Butter (4 tbsp.)
- Swerve or your favorite sweetener (1.5 cups)
- Eggs (4)
- Vanilla (1 tsp.)
- Sour cream (.25 cup)
- Almond flour (1 cup)
- Coconut flour (.25 cup)
- Baking powder (1 tsp.)
- Salt (.25 tsp.)
- *Also Needed*: 12-count muffin tin

Directions for Preparation:

1. Heat the oven to reach 350° Fahrenheit. Prepare the muffin cups with paper liners.

2. Use an electric mixer to cream the butter and sweetener until creamy smooth. Fold in the vanilla and sour cream. Continue mixing, adding the rest of the eggs, one at a time.

3. Stir in both of the flour options, salt, and baking powder. Blend well.

4. Pour the batter into the cups.

5. Bake for 20–30 minutes until they are golden brown.

6. Cool completely and store in the fridge.

ADELE GLENN

61. *Zucchini Chocolate Cake*

Serving Yields Provided: 10

Macro Counts - Each Serving:

- Net Carbs: 7.4 g
- Protein: 10.1 g
- Total Fats: 26.5 g
- Calories: 306

Ingredients Needed:

- Almond flour (3 cups)
- Baking soda (1 tsp.)
- Coconut flour (.25 cup)
- Cacao powder (.5 cup)
- Eggs (4)
- Vanilla extract (3 tsp.)
- Apple cider vinegar (1 tbsp.)
- Melted cacao butter (.25 cup)
- Coconut cream (.75 cup)
- Grated zucchini (2 cups)
- Non-GMO erythritol, birch xylitol, or a blend such as Lakanto (6 tbsp.)
- Salt (1 pinch)

Directions for Preparation:

1. Heat the oven in advance until it reaches 350° Fahrenheit.
2. Prepare the pan with baking paper or a spritz of coconut oil or ghee.
3. Combine the dry components and toss with the rest fixings until combined.
4. Dump the batter into the cake tin.
5. Bake it until it is no longer wobbly in the middle (for 30 to 40 min.). Test the cake for doneness with a cake tester or a sharp knife.
6. Cool it completely and serve plain or with whipped coconut cream, berries, or a simple chocolate glaze.

CHAPTER 8:

21-Day Special Meal Plan for Busy People

Each of these recipes has the net carbs per serving posted. You will see how flexible the plan is when you look at how easy it is to use the recipes in this cookbook for 21 full days, including three meals, snacks, and desserts.

The meals are planned, so you still have flexibility in your eating patterns with extra carbs to use as desired. Even on the strictest diet plan, most of these recipes should be just what the doctor ordered. You have plenty of extra choices, so just enjoy.

Calculate how many carbs you are allowed each day, and add some healthy snacks or sides to the carb count. It's all up to you; just track everything.

Day 1:

Breakfast: Blueberry Flaxseed Muffins: 8.78 grams

Lunch: Egg Salad: 1.4 grams

Dinner: Mongolian Beef: 1.99 grams

Snack or Dessert: Stuffed Mushrooms: 3 grams

Day 2:

Breakfast: Eggs & Sausage Breakfast Sandwich: 6 grams

Lunch: Jalapeno Popper Chicken Salad: 0 grams

Dinner: Stuffed Pork Tenderloin on the Grill: 3 grams

Snack or Dessert: Creamy Lime Pie: 4.2 grams

Day 3:

Breakfast: Pulled Pork Hash: 8 grams

Lunch: Simple Red Cabbage Salad: 0.2 grams

Dinner: BBQ Flank Steak: 1 gram

Snack or Dessert: Pumpkin Caramel Bundt Cake: 5 grams

Day 4:

Breakfast: Smoothie in a Bowl: 4 grams

Lunch: Sloppy Joes – Vegan: 8.9 grams

Dinner: Chicken BBQ Zucchini Boats: 9 grams

Snack or Dessert: Vanilla Shortbread Cookies: 1 gram

Day 5:

Breakfast: Green Buttered Eggs: 2.5 grams

Lunch: Chicken BLT Salad: 4 grams

Dinner: Hamburger Stroganoff: 6 grams

Snack or Dessert: Chocolate Chip Cookie Cheesecake Bars: 5 grams

Day 6:

Breakfast: Cinnamon Raisin Bagels: 6 grams

Lunch: Chicken 'Zoodle' Soup: 4 grams

Dinner: Carnitas – Crockpot: 4 grams

Snack or Dessert: Peanut Butter Fudge: 6 grams

Day 7:

Breakfast: Porridge: 5.4 grams

Lunch: Avocado & Salmon Omelet Wrap: 5.8 grams

Dinner: Barbacoa Beef – Kitchen robot: 2 grams

Snack or Dessert: Raspberry Ice Cream: 3 grams

Day 8:

Breakfast: Belgian Style Waffles: 3 grams

Lunch: Vegetarian Club Salad: 5 grams

Dinner: Baked Tilapia With Cherry Tomatoes: 4 grams

Snack or Dessert: Vanilla Sour Cream Cupcake: 2 grams

Day 9:

Breakfast: Creamy Basil Baked Sausage: 4 grams

Lunch: Warm Peach Scallops Salad: 7 grams

Dinner: Nacho Skillet Steak: 6 grams

Snack or Dessert: Brownie Mug Cake – Kitchen robot: 1.3 grams

Day 10:

Breakfast: Almond Coconut Egg Wraps: 3 grams

Lunch: Chicken Chowder – Crockpot: 7.5 grams

Dinner: Lemon Shrimp: 2.5 grams & Arancini – 5-Cheese Bacon & Cauliflower Bites: 5.4 grams

Snack or Dessert: Sugar-Free Fudgesicles: 1.6 grams

Day 11:

Breakfast: Biscuits & Gravy: 2 grams

Lunch: Greek Salad: 8 grams

Dinner: Cheeseburger Calzones: 3 grams

Snack or Dessert: Keto Magic Bars: 4.5 grams

Day 12:

Breakfast: Pesto Scrambled Eggs: 2.6 grams

Lunch: Alfredo Shrimp: 6.5 grams

Dinner: Chicken & Asparagus: 4 grams

Snack or Dessert: Cheesecake Pudding: 5 grams

Day 13:

Breakfast: Spinach Quiche: 0 grams

Lunch: Chicken, Feta, & Kiwi Salad: 13 grams

Dinner: Bacon Cheeseburger: 0.8 grams

Snack or Dessert: Raspberry Fudge: 4.4 grams

Day 14:

Breakfast: Keto Hot Cross Buns: 2.1 grams

Lunch: Caprese Salad: 4.6 grams

Dinner: Roasted Chicken & Tomatoes: 5 grams

Snack or Dessert: Zucchini Chocolate Cake: 7.4 grams

Day 15:

Breakfast: Almost McGriddle Casserole: 3 grams

Lunch: No-Cook Chilled Avocado & Mint Soup: 4 grams

Dinner: Enchilada: 7 grams

Snack or Dessert: 5-Minute Peanut Butter Mousse: 3 grams

Day 16:

Breakfast: Chocolate Loaf: 2.32 grams

Lunch: Jar Salad with Tempeh – Vegan: 4 grams

Dinner: Slow-Cooked Kalua Pork & Cabbage: 4 grams

Snack or Dessert: Chocolate-Filled Peanut Butter Cookies: 2.7 grams

Day 17:

Breakfast: Bacon Hash: 9 grams

Lunch: Creamy Chicken Soup: 2 grams

Dinner: Slow-Cooked London Broil: 2.5 grams

Snack or Dessert: Almond & Coconut Cake: 3 grams

Day 18:

Breakfast: Cocoa Waffles: 3.4 grams

Lunch: Lobster Salad: 2 grams

Dinner: Parmesan Crusted Pork Chops: 3 grams

Snack or Dessert: Coconut Almond Bars – Kitchen robot: 2 grams

Day 19:

Breakfast: Pumpkin Pancakes: 4 grams

Lunch: Broccoli Curry Soup: 4.8 grams

Dinner: Crack Slaw – Pork Egg Roll in a Bowl: 5.5 grams

Snack or Dessert: No-Bake Chocolate Fudge Haystacks: 1.5 grams

Day 20:

Breakfast: Almonds & Chips Breakfast Cereal: 3 grams

Lunch: Fish Cakes: 0.6 grams & Chinese Sauce Fried Rice: 4.3 grams

Dinner: Sesame Chicken Egg Roll in a Bowl: 3.3 grams

Snack or Dessert: Cinnamon Vanilla Protein Bites: 4 grams

Day 21:

Breakfast: Bagels & Cheese: 8 grams

Lunch: Tuna Salad & Chives: 1 gram

Dinner: BBQ Pork Loin: 3 grams

Snack or Dessert: Chocolate Mini Cakes: 9 grams

CHAPTER 9:

Tips & Tricks to Control Hunger & Avoid Mistakes

How to Maintain Fat Loss

*R*emain Consistent During Fasting: Regardless of the type of weight loss that you ultimately choose to pursue, it's essential to pick one and stick with it. Attempting an intermittent fast for a few days using the keto diet plan before switching to another program, such as the Paleo diet, before trying out a low-carb approach will only cause your body to become confused. It will hold on to every possible calorie until it figures out what the changes mean.

Remember, fasting regularly and consistently is the surest way to see any of its benefits. Only after your body has time to adjust to your new routine will it then be able to adapt appropriately. It can begin to increase the number of positive enzymes and neural pathways to maximize weight loss using this method.

Consider consistency of the "ace-in-the-hole" of proactive weight loss success.

Maintain Your Self-Control: Intermittent fasting only works if your body goes entirely without food for at least twelve hours; any caloric intake resets the cycle. As such, it is imperative to ensure that you maintain control of your bodily urges if you hope to see real results from this type of approach. Remember, fasting for at least twelve hours will only allow you to eat as you usually would or slightly more than an average meal. It doesn't give you free rein to eat everything in sight. Keeping your appetite in check is a strict requirement for success.

Maintain a Calorie Deficit: While this is true for any diet, it is even more true for intermittent fasting since it can be so easy to overeat in such a way that it negates any benefits you might have felt. Remember, you need to burn 3,500 calories on average weekly to lose one pound each week.

Avoid Junk Food: While intermittent fasting means that you will likely have a little extra caloric room in your diet for junk food if you so choose, trying to eat poorly while intermittent fasting will only lead to failure. While you may technically be able to spare the calories, spending the ones you do have on things that won't stick to your ribs for the long haul is a recipe for disaster. Focus on foods that are high in protein and healthy fats. You will feel full and energetic for more prolonged periods every time. You only have so much time you can eat each day, so make it count.

Take It Slow: If you have never gone more than a few hours without eating, then it's a good idea to start slowly. You can go hours without eating and then build up your tolerance from there. It is important to go slow, so if you experience lots of failures early on, it can be more challenging to convince your brain to get into a pro-fasting mindset in the long term. Once you begin to see real weight loss results, you will notice that it will become easier to persevere; all you have to do is make it to that point, and things will begin to fall into place.

Be Aware Of Your Body's Response: While you will want to monitor how your body is reacting to the intermittent fasting process as long as you are regularly withholding calories, this is especially important during the first month while your body is transitioning to a new way of receiving calories. While you may feel faint, lightheaded, shaky, irritable, angry, or weak for up to a month while fasting, symptoms that persist indefinitely are a sign that something ultimately isn't right. It is essential to be in touch with your body enough to know when it's time to consult a health care professional.

Drink Tons of Water: This doesn't mean merely stay hydrated, which is good advice, regardless. It means you should drink at least a gallon of water each day. It will help you feel full and also ensure your body continues processing toxins normally, even if it is holding onto all of its fat because of the transition that is occurring. This is a good exercise for most people anyway, as roughly 40 percent of adults are in a mild state of dehydration. If thirst remains untreated for long enough, it starts manifesting itself as hunger, so staying hydrated will keep you feeling full longer in two ways.

Plan On Staying Busy: While this is a good suggestion in general when it comes to the final few hours of your fast, it's especially important during your transition period. Having nothing to do but sit around for several hours until you can eat again is a sure way to put your untrained body into a situation where it can't help but fail. Don't let this happen to you. Just ensure your fast will break after a period of constant mental activity, and you will find those last few hours going by much faster.

Get More Sleep & Less Stress: If you are a victim of sleep deprivation, you will understand how stressful everyday life is, even before you begin a diet plan.

You may believe it's too late for you, but it isn't. Your diet plan will work, but you may need to make a few other adjustments.

Chronic stress will increase your cortisol levels—the stress hormone. With that action, your hunger levels also rise. The result is that you eat more and put on weight. It's important to find ways to remove the stress, whether it is decluttering your home or taking a vacation.

Eliminate coffee or other forms of caffeine early in the afternoon, and don't consume alcohol for at least three hours before bedtime. Alcohol will also interfere with your quality of sleep, which is why you wake up feeling tired after an evening of nightclubs and boozing.

Recognize Your Cravings

Sugary Foods: Several things can trigger one's desire for sugar, but typically, phosphorous, and tryptophan are the culprits. Have some chicken, beef, lamb, liver, cheese, cauliflower, or broccoli.

Chocolate: The carbon, magnesium, and chromium levels are requesting a portion of spinach, nuts, and seeds, or some broccoli and cheese. It's important to make sure you keep a healthy count of sodium, potassium, and magnesium in your diet. It is suggested to consume a minimum of two teaspoons daily. However, if you crave chocolate, eat chocolate. You need to make sure you eat 75% or higher dark chocolate. Omit milk chocolate from the diet plan.

Fatty or Oily Foods: The levels of calcium and chloride need repair with some spinach, broccoli, cheese, or fish.

Carbs/Bread/Pasta: You need some nitrogen, which can be remedied by eating high-protein meat.

Eat Healthier Snacks During Your Eating Window

Stock your pantry with plenty of high-quality snacks that you can eat when your resistance is down. When you choose snack items, always be sure to select ones that are low in carbs, so your ketone levels will not be disrupted. If you have a busy lifestyle, pick some of the items in the following list, but always remember to count the carbs.

- *Pork Rinds:* Use these to replace chips and crackers. For example, try Pork Clouds, which has a higher quality but without a lot of the offensive oil content.

- *Pepperoni Slices:* Enjoy them with high-fat cheese products, but keep in mind that these are highly processed. Limit your intake of this, and search for hormone-free meat or organic food, if possible.

- *String Cheese:* Choose the full-fat version without additional fillers.

- *Laughing Cow Cheese Wheels:* Purchase full-fat versions and get *real* cheese when possible.

- *Iced Coffee*: Leave the sugar out of your coffee, and use only full-fat milk or cream. Add a bit of MCT oil powder, which can be purchased as chocolate, vanilla, or unflavored.

- *Stevia Sweetened Dark Chocolate*: If you are not using stevia, make sure it's a minimum of 80% or higher in cocoa content.

- *Cacao Nibs*: You can enjoy the same crunch when used as an alternative to chocolate chips.

- *Sugar-Free Jell-O or Popsicles*: You can purchase this ready-to-go, or you can make your own.

Be Sure the Plan Is for You—Avoid Mistakes

As with other things in your life, intermittent fasting may not be for you. You may need to avoid the restrictions if you are included in these categories:

- People with eating disorder histories

- If you are taking prescription medications, you can have issues on taking them on an empty stomach. If you have diabetes, Metformin may cause diarrhea or nausea. Iron supplements may also cause stomach discomfort. Aspirin may also cause an upset stomach or possible ulcers.

- Individuals with diabetes mellitus: type 1 or type 2

- Individuals who experience a drop in his/her blood sugar levels many times

- People who are underweight (BMI≤ 18.5), malnourished, or have other known nutrient deficiencies

- Pregnant women will need more nutrition for the unborn child.

- Nursing mothers will require more nutrients for the baby.

- Children under 18 need more nutrients to grow.

Other Intermittent Dieting Suggestions

If you have tried the 16/8 plan without success, try one of these options.

Skipping Meals: If you're interested in trying out the benefits of intermittent fasting for yourself, but you have an irregular schedule or are not sure if it is for you, then skipping a meal or two, now and then, maybe the type of intermittent fasting for you. As previously discussed, getting into a fasting routine is vital to see the maximum results for your effort, but that doesn't occasionally mean that fasting doesn't come with some benefits as well.

What's more, once you have tried skipping a meal now and then, you can see for yourself just how easy it is, which, in turn, can lead to more positive changes in the future. With so many intermittent fasting options available, the odds are good that one fits your schedule, so give it a try. What have you got to lose, except for a bunch of unessential pounds?

Alternate Day Diet: This form of intermittent fasting means you never have to go long without food if you don't wish to fast for an extended time. Every other day, you should eat regularly, and on the off-days, you merely consume one-fifth of the calories you usually intake on average days.

The average daily caloric consumption is between 2,000 and 2,500 calories, which means that the regular off-day varies between 400 and 500 calories. If you enjoy exercising every day, then this form of intermittent fasting may not be for you since you will have to limit your workouts on off-days severely. When you first begin this technique of intermittent fasting, the easiest way to make it through the low-calorie days is by trying any the protein shakes listed. It is important to work back to "real" natural foods these days because they will always be healthier than the shakes.

This form of intermittent fasting is all about losing weight. Those who try it tend to average between two and three pounds lost per week. If you attempt the Alternate Day Diet, it is critical to eat regularly on your full-calorie days. Binging will not only negate any progress you've made, but it can also cause severe damage to your body if continued over time.

Crescendo Method: This is a method that is ranked as one method suitable for women since you can begin fasting without irritating your hormones or shocking any part of your body using this technique. This is one of the safest programs for women who utilize a fasting window of 12-16 hours. You can enjoy your meals for 8-12 hours. Space it out for a few days, such as Monday, Wednesday, and Friday. If you have failed other diets, this might be your answer. After a two-week period, add one more day of active fasting to your schedule.

Always Check Your Medications for Compatibility

It's important to inform your doctor about your weight loss program. He/she may prescribe some medicines that make you gain weight.

If you are taking insulin injections in high doses, your insulin can impede weight loss. By consuming fewer carbs, you are substantially reducing the requirement of insulin. Again, ask your healthcare professional before you make any changes.

If you are attempting to lose weight, be aware of other probable medications causing weight gain:

- Oral contraceptives

- Antidepressants
- Epilepsy drugs
- Blood pressure medications
- Allergy medicines
- Antibiotics

Know-How: Test for Ketosis Activity

Maintaining ketosis is an individual process, and you need to be sure you are achieving your goals. The levels of beta-hydroxybutyrate, acetone, and acetoacetate can be measured in your urine, breath, and blood.

You can use a *"Ketonix"* meter to measure your breath. You breathe into the meter. The results will be provided by a special coded color that will flash to show your levels of ketosis at that time.

Measure the ketones with a blood ketone meter. All it takes is a small drop of blood on a testing strip inserted into the meter. This process has been researched as an excellent indicator of your current ketosis levels. Unfortunately, the testing strips are expensive.

Test your urine for acetoacetate. The strip is dipped into the urine, which will change the color of the strip. The various shades of purple and pink indicate the levels of ketones. The darker the color on the testing strip, the higher the level of ketones. The major benefit of this is that they are inexpensive. The most effective time to test is early in the morning, after a ketogenic diet dinner, the evening before testing.

You should use one or more of these methods to indicate whether you need to adjust your intake of foods to remain in ketosis.

When you fast, the hormones in your body will change. The keto plan is similar to this process. You could achieve ketosis in just a couple of days once you have used up all your stored glycogen. It can take a month, a week, or just a few days. It all depends on which type of plan you choose. Your protein and carbohydrate intake will determine the time.

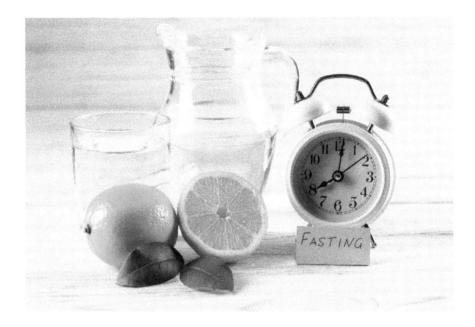

Conclusion

I hope you enjoyed every segment of *Intermittent Fasting*, from the first page to the end, and I hope you can now achieve your goals in weight loss or whatever they may be.

The next step is to gather your essential shopping list and knowledge on the ketogenic diet to travel to the supermarket.

- Prepare the food list consisting of your favorite spices and other products to convert your pantry to keto.

- Begin using your new diet plan, remembering that you can adjust the menu plan using the carbohydrate limitations set for each day. Keep your intake of carbs low.

- Prepare a food journal, and familiarize yourself with an online app to remain in ketosis with ease. You have all of the tools to be successful, but you still need to understand how to test yourself to ensure that you are in ketosis. Your individual progress can be tested using several items to ensure you remain in a ketogenic state. They include testing your breath, blood, or urine.

There is no time like the present to gather your lists of goods needed to begin your ketogenic way of living. Begin with your food and preparation items, and before you know it, you will be stocking your freezer to the brim with all the delicious keto foods your body is craving.

If you find yourself feeling excessively hungry in the early morning hours, the first thing you should keep in mind is that much of this hunger is actually mental, rather than physical. After you have finished the transition, you should notice it much less often. With that being said, it's important to start each day by drinking a liter of water. If you still feel hungry, consider ending your previous day's meal with extra protein and healthy fats which should stick with you through the morning.

Above all, reward yourself. After you have started losing weight, it is important to have a bit of fun. However, you should make sure that it is not a food-related treat. Treat yourself to a massage, or buy a new pair of jeans to show off your loss. Take the family for a game of putt-putt or enjoy a special spa treatment. You deserve it.

While you are considering your reward, why not have a delicious cup of coffee?

This Bulletproof Coffee is for one serving with zero carbs. It has 51 total fats, 1 protein, and 320 calories.

Ingredients Needed:
- MCT oil powder (2 tbsp.)
- Ghee or butter (2 tbsp.)
- Hot coffee (1.5 cups)

Directions for Preparation:
1. Empty the hot coffee into your blender.
2. Pour in the powder and butter. Blend until frothy.
3. Enjoy using a large mug.

Finally, if you found this book useful in any way, a review on Amazon is always appreciated!

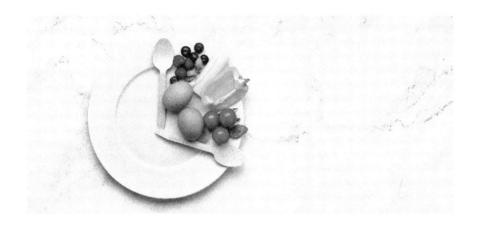

Index For The Recipes:

4. Kale Salad
5. Simple Red Cabbage Salad
6. Tuna Salad & Chives
7. Warm Peach Scallops Salad
8. Vegetarian Club Salad

Soup Choices

1. Chicken 'Zoodle' Soup
2. Creamy Chicken Soup
3. No-Cook Chilled Avocado & Mint Soup

Seafood

1. Fish Cakes
2. Lobster Salad

Other Delicious Lunchtime Choices

1. Mixed Vegetable Patties - Kitchen robot
2. Pesto Roasted Cabbage & Mushrooms
3. Sloppy Joes – Vegan

Chapter 5: Tasty Dinner Choices

Poultry

1. Chicken BBQ Zucchini Boats
2. Roasted Chicken & Tomatoes
3. Sesame Chicken Egg Roll in a Bowl

Pork Options

1. Pan-Fried Chops
2. Parmesan Crusted Pork Chops
3. Slow-Cooked Kalua Pork & Cabbage
4. Stuffed Pork Tenderloin on the Grill

Fish & Seafood Options

1. Lemon Shrimp
2. Skillet Fried Cod

Beef Options

1. Ground Beef Vegetable Skillet
2. Hamburger Stroganoff
3. Mongolian Beef
4. Nacho Skillet Steak
5. Slow-Cooked London Broil

Chapter 6: Snacktime Treats

1. Grilled Zucchini & Cheese Sandwich
2. Pepper Jack Mug Melt
3. Smoked Salmon & Cream Cheese Roll-Ups
4. Spicy Beef Wraps
5. Steak Pinwheels
6. Stuffed Mushrooms

Sweet Snacks

1 Peanut Butter Protein Bars

Chapter 7: Dessert Favorites

1. No-Bake Cheesecake
2. No-Bake Chocolate Fudge Haystacks
3. Peanut Butter Fudge
4. Pumpkin Caramel Bundt Cake
5. Raspberry Fudge
6. Raspberry Ice Cream
7. Sugar-Free Fudgesicles
8. Vanilla Shortbread Cookies
9. Vanilla Sour Cream Cupcake
10. Zucchini Chocolate Cake

CPSIA information can be obtained
at www.ICGtesting.com
Printed in the USA
LVHW071124190221
679465LV00012B/302